Intuitive Eating for Every Day

Intuitive Eating for Every Day

365 Daily Practices & Inspirations to Rediscover the Pleasures of Eating

Evelyn Tribole, MS, RDN, CEDRD-S

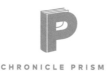

CHRONICLE PRISM

Library of Congress Cataloging-in-Publication Data
Names: Tribole, Evelyn, 1959– author.
Title: Intuitive eating for every day : 365 daily practices & inspirations
   to rediscover the pleasures of eating / Evelyn Tribole.
Description: 1st. | San Francisco : Chronicle Prism, 2021. | Includes
   bibliographical references. | Identifiers: LCCN 2020039491 | ISBN 9781797203980
(paperback) | ISBN 9781797203997 (ebook)
Subjects: LCSH: Weight loss—Psychological aspects. | Food preferences.
Classification: LCC RM222.2 .T7173 2020 | DDC 613.2/5—dc23
LC record available at https://lccn.loc.gov/2020039491

Manufactured in China.

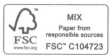

Design by Katie Heit Gardner/Hi, Hello.
Illustration by Marisol Ortega.
Typesetting by Happenstance Type-O-Rama.
Typeset in Mark Pro.

10 9 8 7 6 5 4 3 2

Chronicle books and gifts are available at special quantity discounts to corporations, professional associations, literacy programs, and other organizations. For details and discount information, please contact our premiums department at corporatesales@chroniclebooks.com or at 1-800-759-0190.

CHRONICLE PRISM

Chronicle Prism is an imprint of Chronicle Books LLC,
680 Second Street, San Francisco, California 94107

www.chronicleprism.com

To One and All:

May you flourish and thrive
without oppression.

May you know and own your truth,
experiences, and wisdom.

Here's to being fully grounded
and unshakeable.

CONTENTS

Introduction

Intuitive Eating is a path to personally cultivating a healthy relationship with food, mind, and body. When you can truly honor your internal wisdom and the sensations of your body, you are tapping into a profound strength (dare I say super-power) to get your needs met. Ultimately, the journey evolves into an intimate homecoming anchored in your own unshakeable truth. When you are set free from the tyranny of diet culture, you have more energy and brain space to pursue your passions and purpose. It's nothing short of life changing!

Sadly, most of us have been indoctrinated and immersed in diet culture's messages and rules of eating, which occur at the expense of getting to know our own bodies. This causes confusion and disrupts self-trust because we are looking for the answers outside, when the truest wisdom resides within.

I wrote *Intuitive Eating for Every Day* to help inspire and cultivate connection with your body wisdom. It's not enough to intellectually understand Intuitive Eating, although it's a great start. It takes practice, patience, and intention.

This book of daily practices and inspirations will be your ally and solace against a world steeped in diet culture. It will guide, illuminate, and encourage your Intuitive Eating journey. If you'd like to learn the foundations and unpack the science of

Intuitive Eating, I'd highly recommend you read both *Intuitive Eating*, fourth edition, and the *Intuitive Eating Workbook*.

Intuitive Eating can also be a path to ending the unnecessary suffering of the legacy of diet culture in your family. Through our individual influence and actions, one conversation at a time, we can change the culture.

On a broader level, please keep in mind that if you don't feel safe in your body, it's hard to listen to its messages and wisdom. Ultimately, we need radical inclusivity so that Intuitive Eating can be accessible to all bodies—inclusive of race, gender, sexual orientation, size, abilities, and religion. This means that we need to actively work toward dismantling diet culture and systems of oppression, which perpetuate body shame, weight stigma, racism, poverty, trauma, fear, ableism, and hate. We need more cultural humility, intellectual humility, and life-experience humility, which combined with deep listening, paves the way toward mutual understanding, dignity, and respect for all bodies.

May you have unconditional self-regard.
May you have peace with your body and mind.
May you reclaim and reconnect to the pleasure of eating.
May you be liberated from suffering.

Love, Evelyn

The 10 Principles of Intuitive Eating

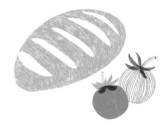

Intuitive Eating is a compassionate, self-care eating framework that treats all bodies with dignity and respect. It is a dynamic interplay of thought, emotion, and instinct rooted in listening to your body's sensations through a process called *interoceptive awareness*. Elyse Resch and I created the Intuitive Eating model described in our original book of the same name, published in 1995. It is now in its fourth edition, and the Intuitive Eating model has more than 125 studies showing its benefits. Here's a review of the ten principles. Please keep in mind that you can't cherry-pick one or two principles and call it Intuitive Eating.

1. REJECT THE DIET MENTALITY

Throw out the diet plans and articles that offer you the false hope of losing weight quickly, easily, and permanently. Get angry at a diet culture that promotes weight loss and the lies that have led you to feel as if you were a failure every time a new diet stopped working and you gained back all of the weight. If you allow even one small hope to linger that a new and better diet or food plan might be lurking around the corner, it will prevent you from being free to rediscover Intuitive Eating.

2. HONOR YOUR HUNGER

Keep your body biologically fed with adequate energy and car-
bohydrates. Otherwise you can trigger a primal drive to overeat.
Once you reach the moment of excessive hunger, all intentions of
moderate, conscious eating are fleeting and irrelevant. Learning
to honor this first biological signal sets the stage for rebuilding
trust in yourself and in food.

3. MAKE PEACE WITH FOOD

Call a truce; stop the food fight! Give yourself unconditional
permission to eat. If you tell yourself that you can't or shouldn't
have a particular food, it can lead to intense feelings of deprivation that build into uncontrollable cravings and, often, bingeing.
When you finally "give in" to your forbidden foods, eating will be
experienced with such intensity it usually results in Last Supper
overeating and overwhelming guilt.

4. CHALLENGE THE FOOD POLICE

Scream a loud "no" to thoughts in your head that declare you're
"good" for eating minimal calories or "bad" because you ate a
piece of chocolate cake. The food police monitor the unreason-
able rules that diet culture has created. The police station is
housed deep in your psyche, and its loudspeaker shouts negative barbs, hopeless phrases, and guilt-provoking indictments.
Chasing the food police away is a critical step in returning to
Intuitive Eating.

5. DISCOVER THE SATISFACTION FACTOR

The Japanese have the wisdom to keep pleasure as one of
their goals of healthy living. In our compulsion to comply with
diet culture, we often overlook one of the most basic gifts of

existence—the pleasure and satisfaction that can be found in the eating experience. When you eat what you really want, in an environment that is inviting, the pleasure you derive will be a powerful force in helping you feel satisfied and content.

6. FEEL YOUR FULLNESS

In order to honor your fullness, you need to trust that you will give yourself the foods that you desire. Listen for the body signals that tell you that you are no longer hungry. Observe the signs that show that you're comfortably full. Pause in the middle of eating and ask yourself how the food tastes, and what your current hunger level is.

7. COPE WITH YOUR EMOTIONS WITH KINDNESS

Recognize that food restriction, both physically and mentally, can trigger loss of control, which can feel like emotional eating. Find kind ways to comfort, nurture, distract, and resolve your issues. Anxiety, loneliness, boredom, and anger are emotions we all experience throughout life. Each has its own trigger, and each has its own appeasement. Food won't fix any of these feelings. It may provide comfort in the short term, distract from the pain, or even numb you. But food won't solve the problem. If anything, eating for emotional hunger may only make you feel worse in the long run. You'll ultimately have to deal with the source of the emotion.

8. RESPECT YOUR BODY

Accept your genetic blueprint. Just as a person with a shoe size of eight would not realistically expect to squeeze into a size six, it is equally futile (and uncomfortable) to have a similar expectation about body size. But mostly, respect your body so you can feel better about who you are. It's hard to reject the diet mentality if you are unrealistic and critical of your body size or shape. All bodies deserve dignity.

9. MOVEMENT—FEEL THE DIFFERENCE

Forget militant exercise. Just get active and *feel* the difference. Shift your focus to how it feels to move your body, rather than the calorie-burning effect of exercise. If you focus on how you feel from working out, such as energized, it can make the difference between rolling out of bed for a brisk morning walk or hitting the snooze alarm.

10. HONOR YOUR HEALTH WITH GENTLE NUTRITION

Make food choices that honor your health and taste buds while making you feel good. Remember that you don't have to eat perfectly to be healthy. You will not suddenly get a nutrient deficiency or become unhealthy from one snack, one meal, or one day of eating. It's what you eat consistently over time that matters. Progress, not perfection, is what counts.

How to Use
This Book

While this book is written as a daily companion with 365 entries, please go at the pace that feels right for you. You might want to linger over some parts and skip others until you feel ready. Overall, the practices and inspirations build on each other, so it's helpful to start at the beginning, but please know that you can revisit any practice at any time.

The process of Intuitive Eating is all about you being the expert on you. There's no way I (or any other person or book) can know your thoughts, experiences, emotions, and background. If a practice seems scary or triggering, it's okay to wait and revisit it later. If you are struggling, you also might want to consider working with a qualified health professional for support (this is especially important if you have an eating disorder, trauma, or a medical or mental health condition). There are over a thousand Certified Intuitive Eating Counselors in twenty-three countries, which are listed in the directory on the IntuitiveEating.org website. There is also a free peer-to-peer support group on the same website, which you may find supportive.

There are fifty-two practices specifically related to the ten Intuitive Eating principles (page 10), which come under the category Weekly Intention. The remaining twelve categories are aspirations and practices that support Intuitive Eating and are summarized in the following section.

Let's first begin with a review of the 10 Intuitive Eating principles:

Principle 1. Reject the Diet Mentality

Principle 2. Honor Your Hunger

Principle 3. Make Peace with Food

Principle 4. Challenge the Food Police

Principle 5. Discover the Satisfaction Factor

Principle 6. Feel Your Fullness

Principle 7. Cope with Your Emotions with Kindness

Principle 8. Respect Your Body

Principle 9. Movement—Feel the Difference

Principle 10. Honor Your Health with Gentle Nutrition

About the Categories in This Book

Here is a brief summary of each of the categories, which are interspersed throughout the book.

Weekly Intentions
Each week begins with a practice of one of the 10 Principles of Intuitive Eating to help cultivate and strengthen the principle.

Midweek Check-In
This is a check-in to see how you are doing with a particular Intuitive Eating practice, which also affirms possible challenges and insights.

Cultivating Trust
Trusting yourself is core to Intuitive Eating. Yet following diet after diet, or food plan after food plan, erodes self-trust and creates self-doubt. These aspirations will help you identify self-trust disruptors and awaken inner knowingness that you and your body can be trusted.

Letting Go of Diet Culture
Diet culture is so seductive. Even when you are clear about its toxicity and harm, it can be hard to let go. This category helps you let go of diet culture by grieving the loss of the fantasies, time, and energy spent on chasing something that was hurtful

to not only your relationship with food, mind, and body—but also to relationships in your life such as a partner, friends, or kids.

Interoceptive Awareness

One of the most profound forms of self-connection is the ability to perceive physical sensations that arise from within your body. This is called interoceptive awareness, which is foundational to Intuitive Eating. Your connection to the physical sensations of your body is a powerful way to recognize your biological and psychological needs.

Consider that every emotion has a physical sensation—from a rapid heartbeat triggered by fear to the jittery stomach flips anticipating a first date. These physical sensations are informing you of your emotional state and possible psychological needs. Similarly, when you experience the pressure from a full bladder or sense the heaviness of sleepy eyelids or hear the rumbling in your stomach for nourishment, your bodily sensations are providing you with powerful messages to get your biological needs met.

Body sensations and perceptions of our senses occur in the present moment. There will be some grounding practices in this section to help connect you with the here and now, which helps you connect with interoceptive awareness. Placing awareness on your various body sensations is like cross-training for Intuitive Eating—it's all interconnected. The more you listen to and connect with the different sensations from your body, the more it will help.

Embodied Affirmations

Research shows that cultivating positive affirmations can be a powerful catalyst for change and also can increase your well-being. To make this more meaningful, I added an embodiment component to help you cultivate a bodily sense and personal connection to the affirming words. Adding this felt sense to an affirmation has made a difference to my patients, and I hope it will for you too.

Self-Compassion
Self-compassion extends an inner kindness to perceived failings and inadequacy. Research shows that self-compassion is a powerful factor in overcoming perfectionism, body dissatisfaction, and alleged eating flaws—which ultimately helps with becoming an Intuitive Eater.

Body Appreciation
Body appreciation is another key factor in cultivating Intuitive Eating and protecting you from harmful diet culture. If you are at war with your body it's unlikely that you would want to listen—let alone respond to its messages and wisdom. This isn't about "loving your body"—it's about appreciating and respecting it.

Self-Care
It's hard to notice the messages of your body when you are burned out or exhausted. Self-care is essential for everyday functioning and thriving in your life—it's about valuing and getting the essentials like adequate sleep, health care, and creating space between projects and meetings. It's a behavioral form of self-kindness—treating yourself as you would a dear friend or loved one.

Meal Meditations
Meal meditations aim to help you cultivate gratitude for different aspects of nourishment.

Emotions and Cravings

Sometimes food cravings are about emotional cravings or unmet needs. All too often, we repress, minimize, or deny the existence of our emotions. But in order to manage emotions, you need to be able to feel them. These reflections and practices will help you get clarity.

Loving Boundaries

In order to get your needs met, it's important to set loving boundaries, which is communicating how you want people to treat you. Setting and maintaining boundaries is a way of taking care of your mental, emotional, and physical health. It's also an important life skill to prevent diet culture from entering your space.

Intuitive Eating Mantras

These are pithy statements to help remind you of the qualities of the Intuitive Eating path and process.

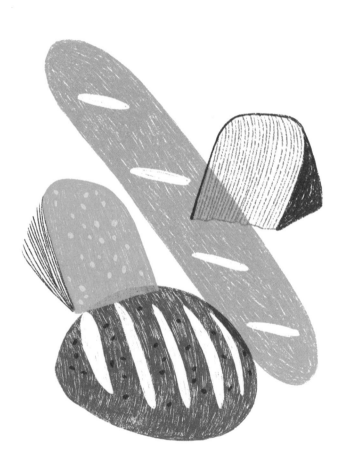

Reject the Diet Mentality

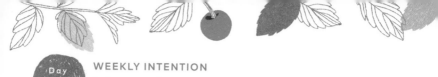

WEEKLY INTENTION
I Spy Diet Culture

Diet culture is very sneaky. It keeps rebranding itself under the guise of wellness, lifestyle, or health. The problem is that whatever names diet culture hides under, its roots remain the same: the perpetuation of fat phobia, body shame, and self-disconnection. To opt out of diet culture, it's important to be able to recognize it. Only through awareness can meaningful change take place.

This week: Set your intention to recognize and *mentally* call out diet culture everywhere you see and hear it. It's akin to the child's game I spy. Consider these sources: conversations with friends, coworkers and family; radio, podcasts, social media, television, movies, places of worship, gyms, hair salons, nail shops, health-care facilities, classrooms, commercials, ads, small talk with strangers, grocery stores.

Calling out diet culture is not about judging other folks. Rather, it's about noticing its ubiquity. Moreover—notice how it makes you feel about your body, eating, and overall state of being.

Day 2

The First Step Is an Act of Trust

Taking the first step on the path of Intuitive Eating is an act of self-trust. It's completely normal to feel wobbly and doubtful. Try not to compare your process to that of others. Each person has their own unique history, with different contributing factors like family of origin, length of time spent dieting, body loathing, and so forth. Consequently, each person will have a different timeline for cultivating a healthy relationship with food, mind, and body.

This is an inward journey of self-connection and healing. It involves a process of unlearning and learning, self-discovery, and growth. In the beginning, it can feel like a leap of faith. That's completely normal.

INTEROCEPTIVE AWARENESS

Deep Listening to the Language of Your Body

Physical sensation is the language of your body—it is constantly communicating with you, whether you are aware of it or not! At first, listening to your body can feel similar to entering a crowded party with lots of noise. As you walk in, there is no discernible conversation, just the ambiguous rumbling sounds of many simultaneous conversations. Yet upon recognition of a familiar face, you say hello and begin talking. It initially takes focused concentration to hear what the other person is saying, but soon the words become clear, and the hum of background chatter seems to fall away. This process is so automatic for most people that they are not usually aware of the focused tuning-in required. This is something you already know how to do. Really! The challenge is the practice of placing your attention on your body sensations.

Day 4

MIDWEEK CHECK-IN

What Have You Noticed About Diet Culture So Far?

When you hear diet culture language or see diet culture behavior, how does it impact you? Does it trigger comparison? Perhaps it makes you mad or anxious? Does it create self-doubt? There's no right or wrong way to feel. Just notice.

BODY APPRECIATION
Your Body Is Your Home

You are not a body—rather you *have* a body, which houses your consciousness, your soul, your spirit, your life force (use whatever descriptor resonates with you). What if you viewed your body as your home for the rest of your life? Every cell in your body is truly part of your one and only home. You don't have to like your home, but it's important to respect it and treat it with dignity. What kind of home environment cultivates loving kindness for yourself and makes you feel welcome? What interiors might need rearranging—perhaps how you talk to yourself? Perhaps how you treat yourself?

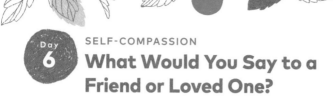

SELF-COMPASSION

What Would You Say to a Friend or Loved One?

The manner in which you speak to yourself has a profound impact on your state of mind. Self-compassion is a vital tool to help cultivate a kind and understanding attitude toward yourself. This perspective-taking helps you quiet the inner bully of internalized diet culture. One way to access self-compassion is to ask yourself, what would you say to a dear friend or loved one in this particular situation? If you are a parent, what would you say to your child?

PRACTICE
If you find your inner bully evoking harsh criticisms and judgment, what would you say to a dear one in this situation?

LETTING GO OF DIET CULTURE

Leaving Diet Culture Doesn't Mean You Are Letting Go of Your Health

People often fear that leaving diet culture behind means abandoning health. Quite the opposite is true! The pursuit of weight loss leads to unhealthy outcomes like weight cycling, binge eating, weight stigma, body dissatisfaction, and increased risk of eating disorders. Similar deleterious outcomes also occur in the context of rigid "healthy" eating. Don't forget that mental health is a foundational part of your overall health. Worrying and stressing about everything you eat is not nourishing for your mind or body.

There's nothing wrong with wanting to feel good. It's possible to pursue sustainable healthy behaviors like getting enough sleep, engaging in joyful movement, and cultivating meaningful relationships. When you let go of the quest (obsession for some) for yet another diet or food plan, you'll actually have more time for other health-promoting pursuits. Remember, weight is not a behavior.

WEEKLY INTENTION

How to Spot Fake Intuitive Eating

With the growing Intuitive Eating movement, many weight loss companies are changing their marketing strategies to capitalize on its popularity. Don't be fooled—they are still rooted in diet culture. A diet is a diet, no matter what you call it. The following are signs of a diet, dressed up in anti-diet language:

- It says it's a psychology-based, science-based, or mindful-eating-based program, BUT it has you counting calories, points, macros, or food groups.

- It lets you eat whatever you want during a specific period of time, BUT you are not allowed to eat outside of that arbitrary time frame, even when you are hungry!

- It's a medically supervised program that has you eliminating food groups, calories, or macros for the sake of shrinking your body. (Sadly, diet culture has hijacked health care too.)

- Before and after pictures are promoted and endorsed as "evidence" of the program working.

- It promotes the idea that weight loss leads to happiness and health.

- It has cheat days.

- It defines "working" by the narrow definition of weight, shape, or size.

This week: Set your intention to notice the varied ways that weight loss programs are sneakily marketed. Include social media, talk shows, advertisements, and friends following such regimens. This practice is to heighten your awareness.

Day
9

INTUITIVE EATING MANTRAS

Intuitive Eating is a journey of one—only I can know what my body needs.

Day
10

SELF-CARE

Self-Renewal as an Act of Self-Kindness

Self-care is about renewal and restoration, which is not self-indulgent. It's about recharging your battery, and getting your basic needs met, so you feel energized and balanced—whether it's for work, school, or helping others. It's hard to listen, let alone respond, to the messages from your body when you are exhausted, depleted, and stressed. Some of the most vital self-care activities are free and mundane, simple essentials—such as getting enough rest or participating in a spiritual practice.

Day 11

MIDWEEK CHECK-IN

Have You Spotted Any Stealth Diet Culture Messaging?

Did you notice any programs, services, social media posts, or ads that co-opt the language of Intuitive Eating, science, mindfulness, or psychology? The key is to get curious and question this messaging, and spot dieting behaviors like counting macros or calories, eliminating food groups, and anything that has you disregarding the needs of your body.

Day 12

LOVING BOUNDARIES

The Importance of Setting Boundaries

Boundaries, or setting limits with other people, are essential for healthy relationships with others *and* yourself. They protect your precious resources, including your time, energy, emotional health, and physical health. Boundaries are also an important tool in moving away from and letting go of diet culture.

Feeling overcommitted, resentful, triggered, spent, or on the verge of burning out are signs that you are giving too much at the expense of you own well-being. How might boundary-setting be supportive here? What would that look like in your own life?

EMBODIED AFFIRMATIONS

Hand on Heart—Intensify

Affirmations are statements about yourself that assert a positive quality, strength, or value that exists within you (even if you don't quite believe it yet!). A body of research shows that there are significant benefits to cultivating positive affirmations, including increased well-being and the rewiring of your brain for positive self-regard.[1]

To get the most out of affirmations, it's helpful to embody them in this way:

1. *Place your hand on your heart.* This nurturing action releases oxytocin, which is a health-promoting natural hormone that confers antistress effects, healing, and the feeling of connection.

2. *Visualize and intensify the positive feeling that you are experiencing.* I'll guide you through the process in the following section.

PRACTICE

Let's try this affirmation: "I am loveable." Place your hand on your heart. If you find it helpful, you may close your eyes for the next step. Recall a situation, a person, or a thing that made you feel loved and safe. Call it to mind, clearly, and focus on the feeling. When this situation is clear in your mind, place your awareness on the felt sense of feeling loved.

Connect with this felt state and, with your hand still on your heart, slowly repeat three times: *I am loveable.*

Day 14

When Were You Told That Your Body Cannot Be Trusted?

You were not born thinking that your body is unreliable or unworthy. Self-trust is interrupted each time you start a diet. If you were put on a diet at a young age, this violation of trust is rooted more profoundly. Trust is broken over and over, each time you deny your body's hunger. This creates doubt and, over time, confusion. Know that every time you connect with your body, you are rebuilding sacred self-trust.

WEEKLY INTENTION

Curate Your Social Media Feeds

The proliferation of picture-perfect posts of foods, photoshopped bodies, and Facetuned selfies on social media can easily trigger the diet mentality and body comparison. One of the best things you can do for yourself is to unfollow any accounts that spark guilt or shame about eating or your body. This also applies to accounts that reinforce harmful fear-mongering messages about health.

This week: Explore accounts that are supportive and uplifting, that promote food freedom and body peace. Look for body positive accounts that feature diverse shapes, sizes, genders, ages, abilities, races, and ethnicities. To help get you started, check out the following Instagram accounts:

@iamlshauntay

@benourishedpdx

@napministry

@bodyposipanda

@eathority

@bodyimage_therapist

@laurathomasphd

@diannebondyyogaofficial

@thebodyisnotanapology

@dietitiananna

@thebodypositive

@foodheaven

@beauty_redefined

@iamchrissyking

@thephitcoach

@foodpeacedietitian

@thetrillrd

@heytiffanyroe

@the_queer_counselor

@i_weigh

@yrfatfriend

@drrachelmillner

@decolonizing_fitness

@allgendernutrition

@ragenchastain

@thefatphobiaslayer

Day 16

Welcome Your Emotions Like Unexpected Guests

In Rumi's classic poem "The Guest House," the Sufi poet suggests that we invite in every emotion like an unexpected visitor, because they are powerful guides. Indeed, imagine the possibilities if we were to greet and welcome all our emotions, as they are portals into identifying our needs. They are the energetic conduit to true self-knowing. Yet, all too often, we bypass the emotions we don't like, while trying to cling to the emotions we enjoy.

The perpetual pursuit of food plans and trying to change your body size rob you of truly getting to know yourself and your emotions. Dieting can serve as a coping mechanism, as can over-exercising—which ultimately disconnects you from your feelings.

Negative emotions can transcend into a wisdom quality—but you need to feel them for that to happen. For example:

- *Loneliness* transcends into valuing meaningful connections and finding ways to cultivate them.

- *Sadness* from loss leads to deeper appreciation of the present moment and not taking relationships for granted.

- *Anger* can become the energizing fuel you need to ask for that raise or set boundaries.

The idea of *feeling your feelings* may sound incredibly vulnerable and daunting. You don't need to fully immerse yourself in your emotions. You can be with them as tolerated, little by little. It's okay to take time-outs, and it's best if you can practice with awareness and intentionality. If you are struggling, it also might be helpful to speak with a therapist who is also trained in Intuitive Eating.

Day 17

INTUITIVE EATING MANTRAS

My body needs to be nourished unconditionally, regardless of what I ate yesterday.

Day 18

MIDWEEK CHECK-IN

Diversify Your Media Feed and Podcasts

Have you explored any new Instagram accounts? When you surround yourself with positive and diverse imagery, free from diet culture, you may start to notice a shift in how you are feeling. How does it feel to be less inundated with diet culture messages? Bonus option: I'd highly recommend giving a listen to these podcasts: *Food Psych* by Christy Harrison, *Food Heaven* by Wendy Lopez and Jessica Jones, *Don't Salt My Game* by Laura Thomas.

INTEROCEPTIVE AWARENESS

Day 19

Attend to Your Body, Like You're Expecting an Important Text Message

We tend to be so vigilant about checking our cell phone multiple times a day. A familiar text notification sound will pull you out of what you are doing. If it's something important, you might drop everything just to respond. What if you viewed your body sensations like personal biological text messages? What if you kindly offered your body that same level of attentiveness—just checking in for physical messages that might need your attention?

LETTING GO OF DIET CULTURE

Day 20

What Is Your Why?

A valuable practice is to reflect on why you want to let go of diet culture (beyond the fact that dieting doesn't work). Becoming crystal clear on your *why* helps you resist getting sucked back into the next latest and greatest diet/lifestyle/food plan, by whatever name it is called. Perhaps you connect with one of these:

- I want my life back.
- I want to be fully present in my here-and-now life.
- I want to end my food and body anxiety.
- I want food and body freedom.
- I want to stop the legacy of diet culture in my family.
- I want to stop the food obsession.
- I want to end being consumed by food guilt and body shame.

Day 21

SELF-COMPASSION

Three Key Steps to Self-Compassion

There is a simple framework developed by self-compassion expert Kristin Neff, PhD, which can help cultivate self-compassion:

1. *Ouch! Acknowledge the moment of suffering, no matter how small.* This can include your self-talk, behaviors, emotions, or situations that cause pain.

2. *Affirm that suffering is part of life.* You are not alone in your suffering. It's normal to struggle.

3. *Say something kind to yourself.* This can include statements that begin with May I_____

   - Be kind to myself.

   - Be patient with myself.

   - Accept myself.

   - Forgive myself and let go of my mistakes.

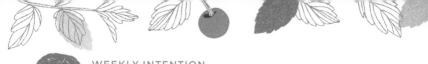

WEEKLY INTENTION

Letting Go of Food Weights and Measures

Many diet programs, a.k.a. lifestyles or food plans, require you to weigh and/or measure your food. Unless you are using a recipe or have a specific medical condition, there really is no need for weights and measures. Your body is not a machine, and it is worthy of your trust.

This week: Reflect on the foods that you might routinely measure—such as cereal, nuts, meats, oils, spreads, and beverages. Think about subtle measurements too, like using your hands as a portion-control monitor. What food or foods could you let go of measuring this week?

Day 23

MEAL MEDITATIONS

May I Nourish Every Cell

I thank my body for all it has allowed me to do today.
I appreciate every cell that works tirelessly for my existence,
From my beating heart cells to breathing lung cells.
May I nourish every cell, in every organ, to complete satisfaction.

BODY APPRECIATION

Create a Personal
I Am More Than a Body Mantra

You were not put on this earth to be gazed upon and objectified; that is not your life's purpose as a human being. You are so much more than a body. Focusing on your physical attributes and comparing your body to others is a form of self-objectification, which is a fast track to unhappiness. You are not alone in this dilemma, as it's a culturally sanctioned form of objectification that perpetuates the internalization of weight stigma.

With unrelenting body commentary by others, you begin to fuse your identity and self-worth with appearance, rather than with who you are as a person. This becomes an automatic thought process, which, if left unchecked, defines you. A helpful step is to remind yourself, repeatedly, that you are so much more than a body. You might also create your own personal mantra; perhaps one of these feels right to you:

- I am more than a body.

- My body does not define my worth.

- My body has nothing to do with my character strengths.

- My body is my home for the rest of my life.

MIDWEEK CHECK-IN

What Weights and Measures Have You Let Go?

If you have been measuring foods for a long time, this might feel daunting. That's okay. It's perfectly fine to go at your own pace. You don't have to let go of everything at once. Perhaps start with one food, one meal, or one snack. With time and repetition, this will get easier.

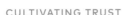

Day 26

CULTIVATING TRUST
Noticing Your Body at Work

Noticing is a powerful practice. Get curious and notice your body working on ordinary activities that we often take for granted. Notice:

- *Your body breathing.* Place your awareness on your lungs. Notice your breath coming in and the breath going out. Notice that you can control your breathing, if you wish.

   Contemplate: How does your body know how to breathe?

- *Your heart beating.* Place your fingers on your wrist and find your pulse. Notice each rhythmic beat.

   Contemplate: How does your body know how to pump blood with its heart?

- *Your eyelids blinking.* Notice that you can control your blinking.

   Contemplate: How do your eyelids know how to blink?

- *Your bladder when it is getting full.* Notice that you can choose when to pee.

   Contemplate: How does your body know how to pee?

Cultivating awareness of your working body helps build connection, confidence, and trust that your body knows how to regulate itself, including knowing when it needs to eat.

INTUITIVE EATING MANTRAS

I choose foods
that satisfy and feel
good in my body.

EMBODIED AFFIRMATIONS

Day 28

I Am Loveable Self-Hug

This technique is known as a self-hug or butterfly hug. This nurturing action also releases oxytocin. Place each of your hands on your opposite arm or shoulder (your arms will be crossed).

How does that feel to you? How does it compare to placing your hand on your heart? There is no wrong or right preference.

PRACTICE

Let's try the butterfly hug with the affirmation "I am loveable." Take a relaxed, seated position and place each of your hands on your opposite shoulder. Recollect a specific time when you felt loved. (It's okay to think about a situation or thing that activated the feeling of being loved—such as an event, a person's actions or words, or a beloved pet.) When this situation is clear in your mind, place your awareness on the felt sense of feeling loved.

Using this felt state, with your hands in a butterfly hug, slowly repeat three times, "*I am loveable.*"

WEEKLY INTENTION

Are You Ready to Delete Tracking Apps?

Part of becoming an Intuitive Eater is to shift your focus to the sensations arising from within your body to guide eating decisions. Outsourcing your eating decisions to an app or tracker disconnects you from your body, which creates doubt. Apps know nothing about your body's needs, preferences, and hunger. Research suggests that these tracking apps are associated with developing and maintaining eating disorder behaviors.[2]

This week: What would it be like to give yourself full permission to delete food and fitness tracker apps? If that feels like too big of a step, how about noticing (with nonjudgmental awareness) how using these apps make you feel?

SELF-CARE

Day 30 Little Acts of Self-Care

What's one easy self-care activity that you can engage in today that will leave you feeling a little bit more restored? Perhaps you can

- Take a 15-minute time-out to close your eyes.

- Ask your partner or roommate to make or pick up dinner.

- Get to bed a little earlier tonight.

- End work on time, rather than working late.

- Choose a bath rather than a shower, for a little more relaxing downtime.

- Watch a sunset.

- Watch the sunrise.

Day 31
"No" Without Explanation Is a Boundary

One of the most straightforward ways to set a boundary is to simply say no, without explanation, to a request. You are not a child. You are not obligated to explain. This might feel really difficult, especially if you tend to be a people pleaser.

Try any of these:

1. No.

2. I would love to, but I can't.

3. No, I wish I could (only state that last part if it resonates with your situation).

4. I'm so disappointed that I need to decline.

5. No, but thank you for thinking of me.

Day 32
What Have You Noticed about Tracking Apps?

Were you able to delete your tracking app? If so, how did that feel? If not, did you notice how using apps to monitor your eating makes you feel? A next step could be simply not using your app, even for just one meal or day at a time.

INTEROCEPTIVE AWARENESS

Day **33**

The Universal Attunement Question

The ability to listen for body sensations can be a daunting idea if you have been disconnected from your body. So many people are living just from their neck up—caught up in the rules of their mind, at the expense of not really knowing how they feel.

Developing interoceptive awareness is about shifting your attention inward. Start now by reflecting on this universal attunement question:

How am I feeling right now—pleasant, unpleasant, or neutral?

It's okay if you are not clear. Simply asking this question and listening for a response is an excellent practice. Notice that this question is not asking what you are feeling emotionally or what level of hunger you are experiencing. It's a broad self-check-in question that connects you with your body. The more you tune in to the experience of your body, the more you will get to know it.

PRACTICE
Pause a few times throughout the day and ask yourself the universal attunement question. Notice how your responses may shift throughout the day.

Day 34
Cost of Diet Culture Harm: Time

It's helpful to get clear about what the pursuit of shrinking your body has really cost you. This is not about judgment, shame, or ridicule. Rather, this process is an emotional inventory, which will serve you on the Intuitive Eating path (especially when part of you wants to try just one more food plan, detox, thirty-day challenge, or whatever name it has).

Reflect on how much time you've spent preoccupied in the pursuit of changing your body. Consider the hours dedicated to preparing food, buying special products, and ruminating over what you are or are not going to eat. How much time would opting out of diet culture give you? Would having this time freed up improve your quality of life?

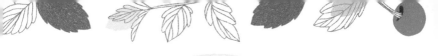

INTUITIVE EATING MANTRAS

Intuitive Eating is a practice of deep inner listening.

WEEKLY INTENTION
Letting Go of Food Labels

A food package has no idea about your level of hunger or the amount of food your body needs to feel satisfied. Yet how often do you let a food label tell you what to do? Using food labels in this manner is a subtle way that you might be using external factors, rather than your body, to guide your eating decisions. What do you do if you are still hungry after eating the arbitrary portion specified on the food label?

This week: Practice letting go of food labels to determine how much you eat. Try eating a few foods this week without looking at the food label.

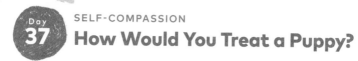

Day 37

How Would You Treat a Puppy?

Self-compassion is more than just how we talk to ourselves; it includes how we treat ourselves. This doesn't come easy when you are used to punishing yourself for perceived "bad behavior," such as violating a food rule. It may help to invoke an image of a puppy as a metaphor. Puppies awaken an innate tenderness and a general knowingness of what to do. You just know that it's best to: Approach it gently. Avoid scaring it. And, of course, never intentionally hurt a puppy. What if we treated ourselves like puppies?

Imagine and contemplate: Notice how you would approach a puppy—do you move toward it, perhaps slowly? How would you talk to the puppy? Do you treat it kindly, even when it makes a mistake?

CULTIVATING TRUST

Repairing Your Self-Trust

Self-trust can be repaired and cultivated. This involves learning to rely upon your inner resources (emotional, cognitive, and physical) to navigate the world, which is very important for psychological health. Think of your body as an integral part of your self-trust navigation system.

Diet culture undermines self-trust and practically beats it out of us. When you are at war with your body or postponing living your life until your body reaches some goal, you are, in essence, living with conditions on yourself.

Self-trust flourishes by what Carl Rogers, founder of humanistic psychology, calls unconditional positive regard for yourself. This means accepting yourself fully—strengths, weaknesses, and all. It's vital for thriving and self-actualization.

The problem is not your body—it's the self-worth, virtue, and identity that culture has projected onto the body. Learning how to accept yourself with unconditional positive regard, simply because you are a human being, is the pathway to freedom.

Day 39

Noticing How Food Labels Impact Thoughts

What thoughts and feelings arise when you check food labels less frequently? Remember that your body has its own inner compass, which helps you navigate hunger, fullness, and ultimately the amount of food that you eat.

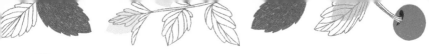

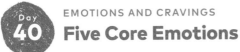

EMOTIONS AND CRAVINGS
Five Core Emotions

Scientists who study emotions mostly agree that there are five core emotions:

anger, fear, disgust, sadness, and enjoyment

Of course, there are many subsets of emotions.[3] The better you get at clearly identifying and truly feeling your emotions, the better you will become at emotional literacy, which ultimately helps you get your needs met. This can be more difficult if you grew up in an environment where you were not allowed to express your feelings, or even were punished for doing so (but it's still possible to learn!).

PRACTICE

As you go about your day, get curious and notice your emotions. Can you identify them? Which of these descriptive qualities would you give those emotions: pleasant, unpleasant, or neutral? What brought this emotion to your awareness? Was it your physical body sensations—such as feeling hot and tense? Or was it perhaps triggered by an event, where you detected a mood shift?

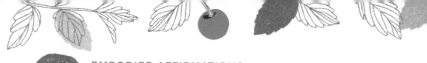

Day 41 | I Am Learning and Growing

It's normal to stumble as you learn new things. It's part of the growth process—not to mention it's very human. Unfortunately, diet culture reinforces perfectionism and all-or-nothing thinking. This practice affirms that the process of learning and growth is paved with fumbles and mistakes, not perfectionism.

PRACTICE

Recollect a situation in which you felt hopeful and proud of yourself because of your progress when learning something new (this can be anything from learning how to play a sport or a new musical instrument, to making a new recipe, speaking a new language, or mastering a new skill). When this situation is clear in your mind, place your awareness on the felt sense of feeling proud. Now intensify this feeling (simply clearly calling it to mind and focusing on the feeling is usually enough to amplify the felt sense of feeling proud).

Using this felt state, with your hand on your heart or in a self-hug, slowly repeat three times, *"I am learning and growing."*

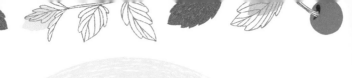

Day 42

INTUITIVE EATING MANTRAS

Nourishing my body
is an act of kindness and
self-respect.

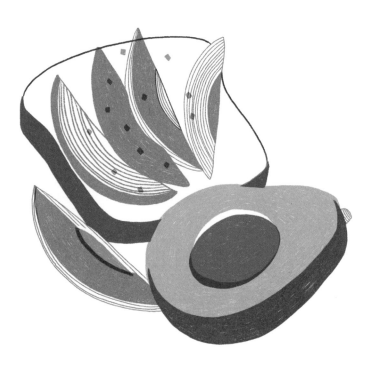

Honor Your Hunger

Day 43

WEEKLY INTENTION
What Are Your First Signs of Hunger?

Your body lets you know that it needs nourishment by exhibiting signs of hunger, which can manifest in different ways for different people. It's helpful to be able to recognize early hunger cues, which are generally a bit subtle. Some people feel hunger through the sensations of a faint rumbling or an empty stomach. Some folks first feel hunger by thinking of food—yes, pleasant thoughts of eating are part of the normal experience of hunger. As the hunger starts to increase, its presence is clearer and sometimes can feel unpleasant. Some folks may experience a shift in mood or a dullness in the ability to focus and concentrate. Others may feel a slight sense of sleepiness or fatigue, even though they had a good night's sleep.

This week: Pay attention to your early signs of hunger. How soon after the signs emerge does it feel best to start eating? What patterns do you see?

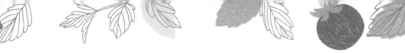

BODY APPRECIATION

Body Appreciation Is Key for Cultivating Intuitive Eating

Appreciation for your body paves the way for a deeper connection, a symbiotic relationship with yourself. It's one thing to hear your body's needs via interoceptive awareness (which is great), but it's equally important to respond to these messages in a timely manner.

A 2017 study on women found that body appreciation was the key mitigating factor between interoceptive awareness and responsiveness among Intuitive Eaters.[4] They were more likely to care for their bodies by granting themselves unconditional permission to eat, relying on internal hunger and satiety cues, and eating for physical rather than emotional reasons.

Day 45
Your Self-Care Is an Important Priority and Is Not Selfish

It's hard to give and be of service to others when your emotional and physical bandwidth is low. That's why it's important to prioritize restoring your vital energy. This shift can be a big hurdle for a lot of people, because they think it's selfish. It's not! Even pilots have mandatory rest periods, because rest is essential in order to perform safely.

This kind of self-care is a necessity, not an indulgent luxury—essential for revitalizing your body, mind, and spirit. These renewal activities tend to be ordinary and accessible, like getting enough sleep (unless you are a new parent!). It can also take the form of setting a time for prayer or meditation.

MIDWEEK CHECK-IN
Day 46
Patterns of Your Hunger

What patterns have you noticed about your hunger signs? Perhaps your hunger begins as a slight sensation in your stomach, then intensifies with a mood shift. There is no right or wrong way to experience hunger. The key is to understand and identify what it feels like for you, in your body.

MEAL MEDITATIONS

Food Is More Than Nutrients and Fuel

May I recognize that food nurtures connections with others.
May I appreciate that food is a shared experience of many traditions.
May I honor that food can both nourish and comfort me.
May I respect that food is a celebration of life.

Day **48**

LETTING GO OF DIET CULTURE

Cost of Diet Culture Harm: Your Peace of Mind Reflection

While in the pursuit of shrinking your body or trying to eat "perfectly" in the name of health, folks often describe their state of mind as preoccupied, humming with background anxiety, or simply just checked out. Has this been true for you?

Reflect on your state of mind when you were dieting, restricting, or following some food plan. Consider what your quality of life would be like if your mind was at peace with food and your body, free from diet culture's toxic grasp. How would it be different?

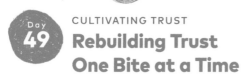

Day 49

Rebuilding Trust One Bite at a Time

Each time you honor your hunger, you are reconnecting with your body and rebuilding trust, one bite at a time. Each bite says, "I got you." Don't ever underestimate this healing act of self-connection.

Fear not, the journey back to your true self is very workable. It will take patience, kindness, and relearning how to self-connect. What perfectionistic tendency or expectation can you let go of today?

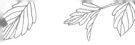
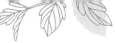

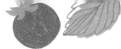

WEEKLY INTENTION
Notice Pleasant Hunger

Most people are familiar with the primal, urgent hunger—the get-out-of my-way, clear-the-decks kind of hunger. I often ask people, "What does pleasant hunger feel like to you?" The most common response is usually a blank stare, followed up by a genuine, "What do you mean?"

Diet culture has demonized hunger as something to be feared or denied, when it is actually a gift—a body cue or physical sensation that alerts you that nourishment is needed. The beginning phase of hunger is generally a somewhat subtle and pleasant experience. You begin thinking about food or looking forward to your next meal—eating sounds appealing. There might be a slight emptiness in your stomach and a rumbling sensation. Or maybe not! The physical sensations vary from person to person.

This week: Set your intention to notice pleasant hunger and how it feels in your body. Notice what you might need in order to recognize this—such as pausing and checking in with yourself. Explore and contrast how it feels to begin a meal when pleasantly hungry, versus feeling the primal, urgent hunger. Which do you prefer?

Day
51

INTUITIVE EATING MANTRAS

The amount and types of foods that *others* eat have no bearing on the unique needs of *my* body.

INTEROCEPTIVE AWARENESS

Day 52

Describe Your Physical Sensation

Body sensations can range from the subtle hunger twang in your stomach to an overt knife-like stabbing pain in your foot from stepping on something sharp. The list of descriptors in the following chart will help you connect to the felt sense in your body. You might want to bookmark this page for easy reference.

LIST OF PHYSICAL SENSATIONS

Texture	Ease/Uneasy	Shape	Movement	Temperature
Bumpy	Clenched	Band-like	Contracted	Burning
Frozen	Constricted	Block-like	Flaccid	Cold
Full	Disconnected	Cord-like	Fluttering	Cool
Gritty	Dull	Crooked	Jittery	Hot
Knotty	Empty	Hollow	Jumpy	Icy
Lumpy	Heavy	Knife-like	Pulsing	Sweaty
Moist	Light	Lacey	Radiating	Temperate
Prickly	Open	Pebble-like	Restless	Warm
Smooth	Numb	Ropy	Stabbing	
Tense	Relaxed	Tubular	Throbbing	**Quality of Sensation**
Thick	Suffocating		Tight	
Tight	Void		Tingly	Neutral
Wooden			Twitchy	Pleasant
				Unpleasant

MIDWEEK CHECK-IN
Discerning Pleasant Hunger

Have you been able to detect subtle, pleasant hunger? This is very nuanced because it takes awareness, willingness, and connection to your body. It might be a while before you hear and recognize the subtlety of pleasant hunger. It can feel frustrating in the beginning, which is completely normal. Remember, this takes practice and time.

SELF-COMPASSION
Self-Compassion Is a Practice

The idea of self-compassion is new for many people. You may love the idea that it's a kind and supportive way of being with yourself. But it's not enough to value the idea of self-compassion intellectually. It's also not enough to view it as important for other people. Rather, it's important to practice it for yourself. If you have operated for most your life with a mind filled with critical self-talk, self-compassion can feel difficult and bumpy in the beginning. Please keep in mind that it's like learning a new language—the language of speaking kindly and supportively to yourself. This takes time.

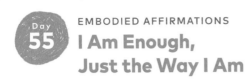

EMBODIED AFFIRMATIONS

Day 55

I Am Enough, Just the Way I Am

Our cultural consumerism conditions us to think that we are not enough and that we need to be fixed and improved upon. Capitalism and diet culture perpetuate and profit from our insecurities.

PRACTICE

Recollect a situation in which you felt that you were enough, just the way you are, with all the qualities that make you who you are at the humanity level. Think about a situation that activated the feeling of enoughness. If this is difficult for you, it may be helpful to reflect on when you were younger. If that is difficult, reflect on being a baby. Babies are precious just as they are—there are no bad babies!

When this situation is clear in your mind, place your awareness on the felt sense of feeling enough. Now intensify this feeling. (Simply calling it to mind, clearly, and focusing on the feeling is usually enough to amplify the felt sense of the feeling, in this case of feeling enough.)

Using this felt state, with your hand on your heart or in a self-hug, slowly repeat three times, *"I am enough, just the way I am."*

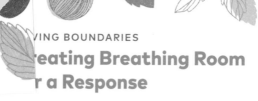

SETTING BOUNDARIES

Creating Breathing Room for a Response

Setting and maintaining boundaries is a learned practice. You might know that you want to decline a project, committee, or an event but feel too wobbly to respond truthfully in the moment. That's okay. A good practice is having some automatic responses on hand to give you a buffer, some breathing room. Try one of these:

- Let me check my calendar and get back to you.

- Let me think about it and get back to you.

- Let me check my work schedule and get back to you.

- Let me check with my family schedule and get back to you.

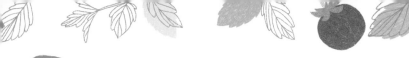

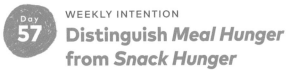

WEEKLY INTENTION
Distinguish *Meal Hunger* from *Snack Hunger*

There are many variants of hunger. Sometimes, people have an unconscious rule that they can only eat a meal's worth of food at meal times. (I like to call this state *meal hungry.*)

It's possible to experience meal hunger at other times of the day for a variety of reasons, such as higher energy needs from significant increase in physical activity—like from playing all day at the beach, or moving into a new home. Or from having a big change in your schedule, like waking up at 5:00 a.m. for an early meeting.

You might eat a substantial breakfast at 5:30 a.m. and be feeling hungry for lunch at 10:30 a.m. Or kids might eat lunch at school at 11:30 a.m., and by the time they play an afternoon sport, they arrive home in a state of meal hunger at 4:30 p.m. These are all examples of hunger as a result of your body working, even though it's not during a traditional mealtime. Just eating a classic snack amount of food will not appease this type of hunger. That's okay! It's normal! Part of the Intuitive Eating journey is learning to honor your hunger according to your body's needs.

This week: Reflect on your hunger levels this week. Occasionally explore this question: Is it possible that I'm meal hungry right now?

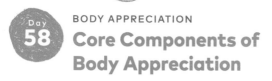

Day 58

Core Components of Body Appreciation

Body appreciation is a practice that helps cultivate Intuitive Eating. Essentially, body appreciation is a protective form of gratitude, which recognizes and amplifies the positive qualities of your body and leads you to honor its needs. Components of body appreciation include

- *Gratitude:* Noticing and being grateful for all that your body can do. This amplifies the positives about your body.

- *Acceptance:* Doesn't mean that you like or love your body. It's like accepting your shoe size or the weather—it just is.

- *Favorable self-evaluation:* Holding yourself in positive regard, which is not based on your body or appearance, rather it's your humanity, values, and character strengths.

- *Caring for your body:* Taking care of your body's needs with nourishment, rest, and self-care.

- *Protecting yourself:* Avoiding the narrowly defined cultural ideal as the only definition of beauty. Rejection of this cultural standard protects your relationship with your precious body.

INTUITIVE EATING MANTRAS

My body does not need
to earn food through
physical activity.

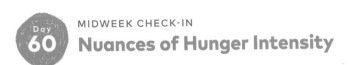

MIDWEEK CHECK-IN
Nuances of Hunger Intensity

Your body is wise and will let you know when you need food.
How are you doing at discerning your various levels of hunger?
Remember that this is not a race, but a practice of awareness.
It's okay if you don't have clarity yet. What's important is that
you are noticing how your body feels with different degrees of
hunger. This process takes time, especially if you have been disconnected for a while.

Day 61

You Are Not Broken

Cultivating self-trust can feel daunting when you've been told most of your life that you can't be trusted with food. For some folks, these messages began in early childhood. For others, it might have begun at puberty, or with some flippant remark from a high school kid or relative or coworker.

Each new diet and food plan erodes self-trust—as they are profound disruptions of getting your basic nourishment needs met. They create a scarcity mentality, both biologically and psychologically, which activates the survival drive to fixate on food. For many folks, this cascade of cellular events triggers binge eating. Dieting and restriction create this response; it is not a character flaw or lack of willpower. Deprivation is a self-trust disruptor.

You have not "failed" the diet—diet culture has failed you. It's understandable with these conditions that you don't trust yourself or your body right now. You are not broken.

LETTING GO OF DIET CULTURE
Cost of Diet Culture Harm: Relationships

Consider the impact of diet culture's eating regimens on your mood (and reactiveness) toward other people—partners, kids, friends, family, coworkers, and others. Perhaps you have been so laser-focused and determined about following your food plan that you've just shut people out and isolated altogether? How has being enmeshed in diet culture affected the quality of your relationships? This can be painful to acknowledge—remember to be kind and compassionate with yourself on this reflection.

Day 63

SELF-CARE
Cozy Sleep Routine

There is no question that adequate sleep is essential for overall well-being and vitality. Sleep deprivation can impact your cognitive capacity, and it wreaks havoc on your hunger and fullness hormones. Stress feels more daunting when you're sleep-deprived.

Juggling life on full throttle can get difficult, and you may reach a point of feeling both wired and tired. A cozy wind-down routine can be incredibly helpful and can become something that you look forward to and enjoy.

- Put on comfortable pajamas.
- Get out clothes and supplies for the next day.
- Turn off electrical devices (cell phone, computer, tablets).
- Relax and reflect for fifteen minutes to an hour, whatever feels right for you.

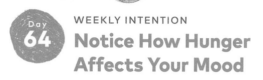

Day 64

WEEKLY INTENTION

Notice How Hunger Affects Your Mood

I love the term *hangry,* a melding of hunger and anger and an apt description of what happens when you wait too long to eat. It greatly affects your mood, impacting the ease of how you move about the world. As hunger builds, there tends to be an increased sense of urgency and impatience, which arises simultaneously with irritability and edginess.

This week: Notice what happens to your mood if you wait too long to eat. Where is that edge for you time-wise? For example, are you perfectly fine mood-wise around three or four hours after eating a meal? Is there a shift toward edginess or irritability around the five- or perhaps six-hour mark after eating? Notice how the quantity of food previously eaten affects your window of irritability. Maybe it's two hours after a snack or five hours after a meal—every body is unique. (Note these time frames are merely prompts, not a rule about when to eat!)

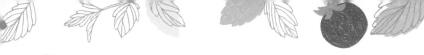

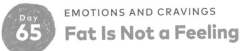

EMOTIONS AND CRAVINGS
Fat Is Not a Feeling

Unpleasant feelings often have a somatic quality of heaviness—which shows up in common sayings like "I need to get this weight off my shoulders" when describing feeling stressed from a burdensome situation. But this is not the same thing as when someone (perhaps you!) says, "I feel fat." There are two problems here. First, feeling fat is not an emotion, although many folks use this language to describe emotional discomfort. This type of thinking is rooted in fat phobia and contributes to weight stigma.

Second, it contributes to confusion about how to get your needs met. Constantly complaining "I feel fat" puts the focus on changing your body and distracts you from the real work (which is often messy and uncomfortable) of figuring out what you really need (such as relationship counseling, a more balanced workload, and so forth). In this scenario, the body becomes the scapegoat and dumping ground for uncomfortable emotions, while perpetuating fat phobia.

It's possible to feel uncomfortable in your body, while simultaneously feeling an uncomfortable feeling, such as anger or disappointment.

PRACTICE
If you find yourself blaming your body for an uncomfortable emotion, unpack what you are truly feeling by asking yourself: What uncomfortable emotion might I truly be feeling?

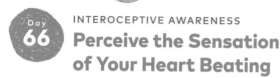

INTEROCEPTIVE AWARENESS

Perceive the Sensation of Your Heart Beating

Can you feel your heart beating without touching your body? This is known as perceiving your heart rate, which is a scientific standard for measuring interoceptive awareness. (Scientists measure this by having folks count their heartbeats, while simultaneously hooking them up to electrodes or a pulse oximeter to directly measure the heart rate.) Unless you are watching a scary movie or being chased by a bear, this might seem like a difficult task. This skill is very nuanced, but I find it makes an excellent interoceptive awareness practice.

PRACTICE

If possible, it's best to set up this practice in a place where you will not be interrupted. Set aside one to five minutes for this practice, whatever feels comfortable for you. When you feel ready, take a quiet seated position.

I find it helpful to warm up to this practice by taking your actual pulse. Simply place your index and middle fingers on the artery on your wrist or the carotid artery on your neck until you reliably and consistently feel the sensation of your heartbeat.

When you feel ready, remove your fingers from the artery and place them comfortably by your side or on your lap. Next, without using your hands, simply perceive your heartbeat. Please be patient with yourself, as this may takes some time. I encourage you to return to this practice, as it's a great way to connect with your body.

Noticing Hunger Irritability

Have you discovered your hangry edge—where you cross over from ordinary hunger to irritability? If you have been honoring your hunger regularly, you won't have this experience—and that's okay too. But sometimes, life throws an unexpected curveball, and you go too long without eating. It's helpful to be able to recognize a mood shift triggered by hunger.

Day 68

INTUITIVE EATING MANTRAS

I eat authentically by honoring my hunger and the satisfaction needs of my unique body.

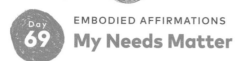

EMBODIED AFFIRMATIONS
My Needs Matter

Being of service to others is wonderful, but it becomes problematic when this comes at the expense of your basic needs. It's hard to connect with others and give of yourself when you are exhausted.

PRACTICE

Recollect a situation in which you recognized that your needs matter. This recognition might have come from an event or situation when you attempted to be all things to all people.

When this situation is clear in your mind, place your awareness on the felt sense of knowing that your needs matter. Now intensify this feeling. (Simply calling it to mind, clearly, and focusing on the feeling is usually enough to amplify the felt sense of the feeling.)

Using this felt knowingness, with your hand on your heart or in a self-hug, slowly repeat three times, *"My needs matter."*

Day 70

MEAL MEDITATIONS

Sacred Time Nourishing Your Body

Thank you for this sacred time to nourish my body.
May this meal be an offering to connect with
my body in a meaningful way.
May I discover the delightful contentedness of *just right* fullness.
May I give myself grace when learning about my body and needs.
May I protect this sacred time for my body.

Day 71

WEEKLY INTENTION

It's Okay to Be Annoyed by Hunger. Just be Prepared.

It's a beautiful thing to honor your hunger. But hunger can also be annoying! That's okay—that's a completely normal feeling. Sometimes hunger is inconvenient. Sometimes it catches you off guard. Sometimes you have hungrier days. An important part of self-care is being ready for those times and responding to your body's needs with kindness.

This week: What types of easy access snacks sustain you and taste good? What do you need in order to have them available, even at inconvenient times and situations?

SELF-COMPASSION

Be Kind to Yourself, Especially When You're Struggling

Talking kindly to yourself when you are struggling can feel like a radical act. Here's a little perspective. If you saw a little kid learning to ride a bike, but she kept falling down, would you yell at and denigrate her? Do you think criticizing her would help her relax and concentrate on the process of riding a bike? Or do you think it would make it harder?

What if you shouted encouraging words such as, "Yes, this takes practice! It's normal to wobble. You are putting in great effort."? Now, could you try that encouraging attitude for yourself as you are learning to self-connect? What could you say?

Day
73

CULTIVATING TRUST
Yet Is a Powerful Mindset, which Builds Trust

The concept of mindset was developed and validated by Stanford psychologist Carol Dweck and popularized in her book *Mindset: The New Psychology of Success.*[5] Her research demonstrates that a growth mindset can be learned. It's a powerful perspective shift reflecting that we have agency (a form of self-trust) and that with consistent work we can develop and grow our basic abilities.

The word *yet* is part of the language of the growth mindset. It acknowledges that you are in process and continually learning.

Read aloud these two statements. Notice how you feel after reciting each statement:

I am not an Intuitive Eater.

I am not an Intuitive Eater, yet.

Did you notice a shift in how you feel when you add the descriptor *yet*?

PRACTICE

Try adding *yet* to some of your self-talk statements. There are many ways to use this. You can try one of these, or create one that better fits your situation.

I have not recognized hunger, yet.

I have not recognized fullness, yet.

I have not let go of diet culture, yet.

MIDWEEK CHECK-IN

The Sometimes Inconvenience of Hunger

Part of the art of living is to be prepared for the sometimes inconvenience of hunger. Were you able to have snacks on hand or nearby? Did it make a difference, such as creating a calming effect, to just know food was around? If preparing for such times has been challenging for you, what might you need to overcome this obstacle? Perhaps you need to build in a little more time. Maybe you need to plan to get to a store. Or maybe you have yet to discover your favorite snacks that sustain and satisfy you. That's okay—this process takes time and patience.

LETTING GO OF DIET CULTURE
Letting Go of Diet Culture Bonding

When you are entangled in the throes of diet culture, it's very common to bond with others over the pursuit of the "perfect" meal plan or workout. It's this type of socially acceptable small talk that often progresses into friendships. What would these conversations and friendships look like without the diet culture talk? Could you have conversations that don't gossip about bodies or demonize foods? What else might you talk about or have in common?

Day
76

INTUITIVE EATING MANTRAS

My Intuitive Eating
journey is my own,
and no two Intuitive
Eating journeys
are the same.

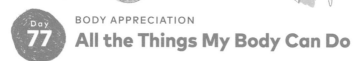

BODY APPRECIATION

Day 77
All the Things My Body Can Do

Wrapping your self-worth in the appearance of your body leads to a host of problems, including unhappiness, body dissatisfaction, and self-loathing. One way out of this self-objectifying dilemma is to shift your focus on the amazing things your body can do—from perceiving sensory experiences to cultivating connection with others.

Take a moment to review the following chart. Reflect on the importance of some of these bodily functions to your life. What do these functions mean to you?

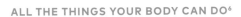

ALL THE THINGS YOUR BODY CAN DO[6]

Sensation

Experience pleasure
Feel emotion
Hearing
Sight
Smell
Taste
Touch

Self-Care

Cooking
Drinking
Eating
Grooming
Sleeping/ Napping

Movement

Agility
Balance
Climbing
Dancing
Driving
Energy level
Exercise
Flexibility
Jumping
Physical coordination
Reflexes
Sports
Walking

Health

Absorb nutrients
Breathe
Create a baby
Digest food
General restoration
Grow (hair, nails, skin cells, etc.)
Heal from a cold
Heal from a wound
Regulate temperature, hunger, thirst, etc.
Remove toxins (through the liver, lungs, and kidneys)

Creativity

Building
Carving
Crafting
Drawing
Gardening
Painting
Photography
Playing an instrument
Reading
Sculpting
Singing
Writing

Connection with Others

Body language
Cuddling
Facial expressions (e.g., smiling)
Giving/ Receiving a massage
Holding Hands
Hugging
Kissing
Making eye contact
Sexual activities
Shaking hands
Shoulder to cry on
Talking

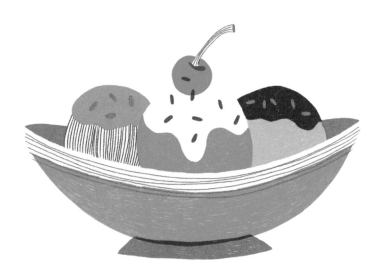

Make Peace with Food

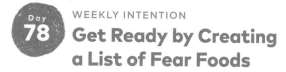

WEEKLY INTENTION

Get Ready by Creating a List of Fear Foods

Making peace with food is about giving yourself unconditional permission to eat whatever food you want, with attunement to how your body is feeling. It's one of the hallmarks of being an Intuitive Eater. For many people, this is the scariest principle of Intuitive Eating. Rather than dive into this principle, let's ease in, by getting your mind ready.

This week: First, make a list of all your forbidden foods. You might find it helpful to do this activity on a sheet of paper, but you can also do this on a computer or note-taking app on your phone. Be sure to include the foods that you allow yourself to eat, but eating them invokes a feeling of guilt or unease.

Next, categorize the foods according to their fear level, and put them in the following chart, *My Hierarchy of Fear Foods*. We will use this chart much later. Contemplate daily: What would it be like to eat and even enjoy these foods without guilt or anxiety?

MY HIERARCHY OF FEAR FOODS CHART

Scary			
Scarier			
Scariest			

LOVING BOUNDARIES

Boundaries about Body Compliments

Handling body compliments can feel awkward, in part because of the attention placed on your body and in part because it is objectifying. You can teach people, kindly, that you do not want these comments and that they can unintentionally cause harm.

Speaking up not only helps yourself, it also creates a healing ripple effect to combat the unfortunate societal norm of commenting on people's bodies. Here's some language that can help in these situations:

"I realize that you were trying to give me a compliment when you said I looked good because I've lost weight. I feel uncomfortable when people comment on my body or the bodies of other people. People on the receiving end of this body comment could have an eating disorder, cancer, or depression—something they might not feel comfortable disclosing."

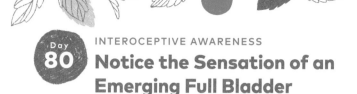

Day 80

Notice the Sensation of an Emerging Full Bladder

How often do you take the sensation of the need to pee for granted? Feeling that your bladder is full is a great example of being connected to the sensations of your body. When I ask my patients how they know when to pee (it's *wee* for the Aussies)— I'm met with a wide variety of reactions from incredulity to laughter. Eventually, there's a nodding affirmation, indicating "Of course I know when to do that!"

We learn early in life what happens if we ignore this important body cue—a very uncomfortable mess, to say the least. It's such a commonly understood felt sense that it needs no further explanation. I find it an easy gateway, an accessible way to help you get more connected with your body—because there is no moral imperative attached to this process, unlike eating with the undue influence of diet culture.

PRACTICE

The next time you need to pee, notice the emerging physical sensation of needing to pee—where do you feel it in your body? Take care to engage in this practice from direct experience in your body, rather than an intellectualized exercise.

MIDWEEK CHECK-IN

Contemplating Your Fear Foods

How are you doing with creating your hierarchy of fear foods? On the one hand, it's a pretty straightforward process and not too hard to create this list. On the other hand, you might find yourself approaching it with a sense of dread and wanting to put it off. Remember, this step is not asking you to actually eat the food. Rather, it's about contemplating what your life would be like to be able to eat these foods without anxiety. Research analyzing the Stages of Change psychology model shows that just contemplating and visualizing what a change would be like is a valid step.[7] It's basically a practice for your mind that gets you ready.

Day
82

SELF-CARE

You Can't Be All Things to All People

We don't think twice about the need to charge our cell phones, especially when the battery is low—they won't work without energy. Similarly, your energy is a vital, limited resource. You cannot be all things to all people. Even if one of your highest values is to be of service to other people, you can't be effective if you are wiped out. Prioritizing getting a full night's sleep, nourishing your body in a timely manner, making time to reflect, and so on strengthens your connection to yourself and others.

I Am Worth So Much More Than What My Body Looks Like, in Shape, Size, or Weight

Diet culture objectifies our bodies, tying self-worth to appearance. This affirmation will remind you that you are far more than your appearance.

PRACTICE

Reflect on all the people in your life whom you love. Is your love for them dependent on their shape, weight, or body size? Of course not! Recollect a situation in which you realized that you are so much more than your body. Perhaps it was a time you were engaged in an act of service, achieved an accomplishment, or experienced a spiritual knowing.

When this situation is clear in your mind, place your awareness on the felt sense of knowing that you are so much more than your body. Now intensify this feeling. (Simply calling it to mind, clearly, and focusing on the feeling is usually enough to amplify the felt sense of the feeling.)

Using this felt knowingness, with your hand on your heart or in a self-hug, slowly repeat three times, "*I am worth so much more than what my body looks like, in shape, size, or weight.*"

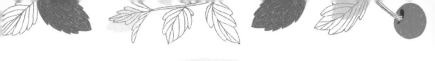

Day
84

INTUITIVE EATING MANTRAS

May I stay connected
with the sensations
of my body.

WEEKLY INTENTION
Viewing Food as a Means of Social Connection

Eating is more than just nourishment—it is a means of social connection. When your list of acceptable foods becomes shorter and shorter, it impacts your eating experiences by increasing your anxiety when your "safe foods" are not available. Broadening your list of acceptable foods by making peace with eating them is the pathway to freedom, flexibility, and calm.

This week: Reflect on the following: How does having restricted food intake or forbidden foods impact your relationships? For example, does it increase your anxiety around others? Perhaps you turn down social invitations because you don't want to deal with the food?

If you were to ease up and allow one food back into your eating repertoire, which food would move you closer to social eating without anxiety—maybe pizza, potluck food, or restaurant food?

CULTIVATING TRUST
Your Body Is Wired to Survive

Losing control of eating is often a consequence of food restriction—both mental and physical. Your cells don't recognize the difference between an intentional food restriction for the purpose of shrinking your body (a.k.a. dieting) and an unintentional one imposed by famine. Since famines have existed since the dawn of humankind, compensatory eating makes sense: It is a vital protection mechanism for survival. Studies looking at the unintended consequences of dieting or food restriction report some form of loss-of-control eating or binge eating.[8]

If you have a history of food scarcity or food insecurity of any kind, it's not uncommon to engage in loss-of-control eating or binge eating as a result.[9]

Shifting your perspective to "I have a very smart body that is wired to survive" can help you recognize that your body is working to protect you. Your body is not broken. You are not broken.

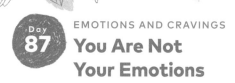

Day 87

You Are Not
Your Emotions

Emotions are powerful forms of energy that, at times, can seem to overwhelm your mind and body. While it might be obvious, it's important to remind yourself that you are not your emotions—especially in turbulent times. Emotions are not your identity.

Just the act of how you describe your emotions can make a difference in how you feel. Try this slight change in wording and observe the space it provides between the emotions experienced and your self-identity. You may notice that you are less likely to get swallowed up and entangled with your emotions.

Instead of	Try
I am angry.	*I feel angry.*
I am sad.	*I feel sad.*
I am disappointed.	*I feel disappointed.*

Day 88

Contemplating Fear Foods That Offer Social Connection

Continue to reflect on how the ability to eat some of your fear foods would increase your social connection. Perhaps it means that at a social gathering involving food, you will be present, rather than distracted and worried about your eating. Maybe it means you will accept more spontaneous invitations organized around food, such as potlucks, a last-minute breakfast with a friend, or appetizers with coworkers.

SELF-COMPASSION

Day 89

Dampening Your Inner Bully and Critic

It can feel painful to look at your self-talk or thoughts when they are mean and nasty. Yet we need to be aware of and uproot this kind of thinking. That's why the lens of self-compassion is so important—it's an inner self-kindness, with a nonjudgmental understanding. It's an essential tool.

When your inner critic starts barking, pause and notice how it makes you feel. Really notice the emotional pain and discomfort. What's a more supportive, warm, and encouraging way to reframe these thoughts? What would you say to a friend or loved one who was in a similar situation with these thoughts?

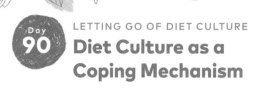

LETTING GO OF DIET CULTURE

Diet Culture as a Coping Mechanism

Life is messy. Sometimes, letting go of diets is difficult because of the subtle but significant role they can play in distracting you from life's inevitable challenges and transitions, such as moving to a new school, going to college, becoming a parent, navigating relationship issues, starting a new job, coping with loneliness, and so forth.

Starting a new food plan gives you a focus, even a purpose, with very specific instructions and hope for the future. The pursuit of shrinking the body temporarily provides a distraction but does absolutely nothing to deal with your real-life trials and tribulations. When the diet ultimately fails you, you are left feeling even worse—betrayed by yet another diet and still facing life's challenges.

Letting go of dieting gives you the gift of living an authentic life and building resiliency for when life throws you a curveball.

BODY APPRECIATION

Day 91

Lean In to Your Values, Rather than Your Body

One way to loosen the stronghold of being overidentified with your body is to shift your focus to the values you hold true. Your core values don't change, but seasons and bodies do.

It's helpful to name your values because they will more easily come to mind, becoming mentally accessible and ultimately more acted upon with your life choices.[10] Reflect upon what really matters to you, deep in your heart. How do you want spend your time on this earth? What sort of person do you aspire to be? If you had to whittle down your values—what are your top three?

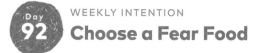

WEEKLY INTENTION

Day 92 Choose a Fear Food

Having flexibility with your eating choices is important for your emotional and social health. Remember, you are not a good or bad person based on what you eat! Let's take an action step and eat one of your fear foods. Refer to your hierarchy of fear foods (p. 88) and consider the following questions (there are no wrong or right answers):

- Would it feel better to start with the least scary food or to just jump right in to the scariest food?

- Do you want to eat the food alone or with other, supportive people?

- Would you prefer to eat the food at home or go out for it?

- What do you need to feel emotionally safe? (For example, you can ask anyone you live with to avoid commenting on your food choices.)

This week: Plan to eat a fear food, either as part of a meal or about an hour or two later (so that intense hunger won't dominate the eating experience). Before you begin eating, notice how you feel. Excited? Worried? Perhaps a combination of feelings; that's completely normal. It can be helpful to ground yourself with a couple of relaxing breaths and an intention: that you are taking a brave step toward healing your relationship with food.

During the experience of eating notice taste, texture, and so forth. Observe any thoughts that arise.

When you finish eating reflect on your experience. Did it meet your expectations? Did anything surprise you? How did you feel when you finished, both physically and emotionally?

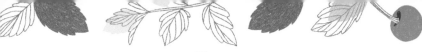

Day
93

MEAL MEDITATIONS

Pleasure and Peace

May I experience pleasure in eating this meal.
May I especially experience delight in the first bite.
May I have peace on my plate and in my mind.
May I eat with ease and joy.

Day
94

INTUITIVE EATING MANTRAS

My Intuitive Eating journey is a process of learning and discovery, there is no failure.

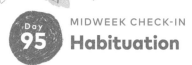

Day 95

Habituation

Have you eaten or planned to eat a fear food yet? This is a big step, and often a very difficult one. It's important to be kind and gentle with yourself. It can be helpful to remind yourself why you are doing this (such as having more freedom or a less fraught relationship with food). If you are anxious about this step, it can be helpful to take a couple of relaxing breaths and do a little grounding practice (see Day 262, Day 275, or Day 286) before you begin eating.

If you have eaten a fear food, do you dread the idea of eating it again? Please know that this is a normal experience in the beginning. It takes many repetitions of eating a forbidden food to take the excitement and anxiety out of the eating process. Scientifically, this is known as a habituation response, where novelty triggers excitement. Conversely, frequent experiences cultivate a no-big-deal attitude toward eating.

Day 96

The Body Sensation of Breathing Practice

Many spiritual traditions have used the breath as a focal point of concentration, such as the practice of yoga and meditation. For your entire life, no matter where you go, you have access to your breath. No technology or special equipment needed.

It will be helpful to set up the following practice in a place where you are unlikely to be interrupted. Set aside one to five minutes for this practice, whatever feels comfortable for you. When you feel ready, take a quiet seated position.

PRACTICE

Take a relaxed, normal inhalation of your breath. Place your awareness on the sensation of your body breathing. Notice how your lungs *feel* filling up with air and the sensation of your chest gradually expanding. As you begin to exhale, notice the sensation of your breath going out, with your chest contracting. Don't worry if you discover that your mind is wandering (perhaps reviewing your perpetual to-do list), it's no problem. Kindly and without judgment, redirect your awareness to the felt sensation of your body breathing.

EXTENDED PRACTICE

Practice feeling the sensation of breathing during natural pauses and waiting periods throughout your day.

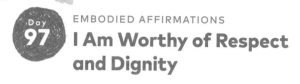

Day 97

I Am Worthy of Respect and Dignity

Diet culture places a hierarchy and morality on body size. It's easy to get preoccupied in the toxic cultural thought process, which leads to automatic self-denigration if you don't match up to the impossible cultural ideal. It's important to remind yourself that all bodies, including your own, are deserving of respect and dignity.

PRACTICE

Reflect upon a time or situation in which you felt worthy of respect and dignity. When this situation is clear in your mind, place your awareness on the felt sense of knowing that you are worthy of respect and dignity, without conditions or performance. Now intensify this feeling. (Simply calling it to mind, clearly, and focusing on the feeling is usually enough to amplify the felt sense of the feeling.)

Using this felt knowingness, with your hand on your heart or in a self-hug, repeat three times, *"I am worthy of respect and dignity."*

Day 98

CULTIVATING TRUST

This Is Your Body Working

Diet culture keeps you in a perpetually underfed state. This means you are simultaneously wanting food and trying to avoid it. It's this frenetic push-pull relationship with eating that undermines self-trust because you are denying your body's basic need to eat, which is no different or less important than the need to breathe.

If you have a history of dieting or following restrictive food plans in hopes of shrinking your body, you likely have experienced episodes of feeling like you can't control how much you eat, as if you are one bite away from a binge. This is your body trying to protect you from what it perceives as a famine.

Think of this: If you hold your breath for a long time, then finally take in your first panicked inhale, no one calls it "loss of control breathing" or "binge breathing"! It's a normal compensatory response to air deprivation.

Part of cultivating trust is accepting your body's need to inhale food as a consequence of food restriction—even if you don't want to. That's a normal response. There is no shame in that. It's important to shift your perspective, that this is *your* body working to protect you.

WEEKLY INTENTION

Eat a Fear Food That Increases Social Connection

It's not uncommon for people to turn down social events because of their fear that off-limit foods may be served. Or other times, they may show up but have incredible anxiety around eating or being near fear foods. Consequently, they are not able to really connect with the people and friends who are important in their life. Instead, they are distracted with the inner anxious chatter of what to eat, what not to eat, and how much to eat.

This week: Practice eating a fear food that would give you more social connection—either because it will lower your food anxiety with these types of experiences and/or it's a socially connected food. Consider these types of foods and situations: sharing a pizza, roasting marshmallows, sharing a bucket of popcorn at the movies, or going out for dessert.

Day 100 Be Kind to Your Mind—Recognizing Activities That Drain You

Mental well-being is an important part of health that is often left out of the conversation. Sometimes you need to take a time-out to refresh your emotional and energetic bandwidth. What types of activities drain your emotional energy?

- Scrolling through social media
- Conversations with a friend that are not reciprocal
- Volunteering for projects that are not aligned with your values or vision
- Your own perfectionism
- Unrealistic expectations and deadlines
- Watching or reading too much news

Which of these activities might you ease up on or set aside for a little mental health break?

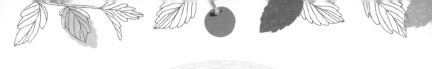

Day
101

INTUITIVE EATING MANTRAS

Intuitive Eating is
an empowering act of
self-connection.

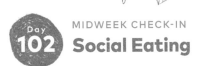

Day 102 Social Eating

Have you made a plan to eat a fear food yet? Perhaps you are still avoiding this practice. Consider choosing to have this eating experience with someone you really trust, and who makes you feel safe and accepted. If you feel comfortable, let them know what you are doing and what you need from them. Perhaps you need them to socialize as usual, but to avoid making any comments about what you are eating. Let them know that sometimes even well-meaning comments like, "I haven't seen you eat dessert in forever," can feel uncomfortable.

LOVING BOUNDARIES

What to Do About Friends Who Are Really into Eating Plans, Cleanses, and So On

When people are down the rabbit hole of the latest diet/food/ wellness craze, they enter a profound self-absorption about their eating. One problem is that they are usually completely unaware. They don't read the cues or body language of the disinterested folks to whom they are espousing. It often goes on ad nauseam because people just don't know how to politely interrupt the dietary monologue.

The best bet is to be direct, preferably having a little chat in private before your next social gathering. You might try saying something like this:

"I know you are very enthusiastic about your new eating plan, but I'm really working hard on healing my relationship with food. I feel really triggered by anyone who starts talking about diets, cleanses, and fasts. I'm wondering if you can support me by not talking about it?" If they answer yes, thank them. Then politely ask how you can remind them of this agreement if they forget, which is really common!

LETTING GO OF DIET CULTURE
Missing the Rush of a New Food Plan

It's very common to feel a little lost and sad when you are letting go of diet culture. This is normal, and it's important to let yourself feel your authentic feelings. You may long for the excitement and rush of hope of starting the new latest and greatest diet or "lifestyle" change.

In these times, it's helpful to remember that your body is smart. Your mind is smart. Your experiences have taught you that diets simply don't work. They are not sustainable in the long run. A body of research also shows that the vast majority of people regain any weight they lost, with up to two-thirds of those people gaining more weight than what was originally lost![11] (Please note that there is nothing inherently wrong with weight gain, but this is a profound paradox given it's the opposite outcome people are seeking when they begin a diet.)

It's normal to feel diet culture's seductive call, but the price is just too big. Once your eyes and experience are opened to the truth, you just can't go back.

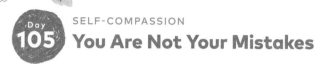

Day 105
You Are Not Your Mistakes

It's really easy to get absorbed in the throes of a situation and overidentify with your emotions or an event. Yes, you may be struggling. Yes, you may have made a mistake. This does not make you a failure. It makes you human, and it makes you resilient—it's how you learn and grow with your experiences.

Personalizing or overidentifying with a situation creates a distortion of your sense of self, which makes it all too easy to get swept away by negative emotions and reactivity. Remember that you are learning and growing with your experiences. Making mistakes is a normal and inescapable part of being human.

WEEKLY INTENTION
Making Peace with a Food Group

Diet culture is like fashion: Without fail, there always seems to be a new hot trend of the latest and greatest diet or villainous ingredient or superfood. Back in the eighties and nineties, fat was definitely out.[12] Now fat seems to be making its way back into the exonerated groups of foods. Because of fickle diet culture, it is sadly common for people to eliminate entire groups of foods such as grains, carbs, or fats.

This week: Choose a food from a group that you are afraid to eat. What food sounds good? What would give you more flexibility in eating? Perhaps bread, so that you can enjoy meals that include sandwiches, french toast, or paninis?

BODY APPRECIATION
Cultivating Your Inner Firewall: Protection from Fat Phobia

Your humanity is precious and deserves protection from the proliferation of fat phobia, which shows up in media, conversations, schools, health care, and social media. Just like firewalls protect computers and websites from malware and viruses, we need an internal system to build resilience against fat phobia. Which of these mantras and actions resonates with you? Pick a couple to use as your inner firewall:

- I do not define my self-worth based on appearance or body size.

- I cannot tell someone's health, fitness, values, or character based on the size of their body.

- I reject any messages that show before and after pictures, which are a form of body hierarchy and objectification.

- Fat phobia is rooted in racism and patriarchy. I don't buy into these oppressive systems. (Note that these toxic systems need to be dismantled, but building resilience in the meantime is a valuable tool.)

- Preoccupation with my appearance is a fast track to unhappiness.

- Reject and unfollow any messages, including on social media, that objectify bodies.

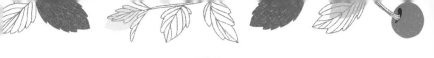

Day
108

INTUITIVE EATING MANTRAS

May I eat without guilt or moral dilemma.

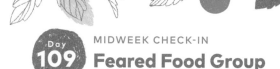

Feared Food Group

How are you doing with plans to eat something from a group of foods that triggers fear? When diet culture has deemed a particular group of food as "bad," it can feel especially challenging to eat these foods, because you are picking up on the collective anxiety and judgment from the culture. Keep in mind that diet culture operates on fearmongering, while perpetuating fads and misinformation. Remember that butter was once considered "bad," and now diet culture has people putting butter in their coffee! The act of eating a fear food moves you one step closer to the liberation and food freedom that we all deserve. That's something to celebrate!

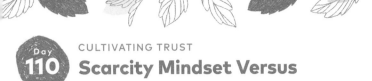

Day 110

Scarcity Mindset Versus Abundance

One of the best examples of the scarcity mindset is when people started panic-buying (and even hoarding) toilet paper during the coronavirus pandemic of 2020. It put people on edge. They were constantly worrying that they would run out of toilet paper. They didn't trust there would be enough, even though there was plenty in the supply chain.

The scarcity mindset creates doubt and lack of trust, whether around toilet paper or food. Just a mere threat of "not having enough" sets in place a hyperfocus and vigilance of "Will I get enough?" That's why dieting and food restriction conditions your mind to perpetually focus on eating. It's a normal consequence. Your mind and body are actually working together to ensure your survival.

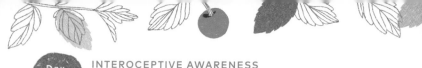

Day 111

Respond to Body Sensations in a Timely Manner

It's not enough to merely hear a body cue or sensation. It's important to attend to it. Responding to a sensation from your body is known as interoceptive responsivity.

How responsive are you to the general needs of your body? When you have the first signs of a full bladder, do you tend to empty it right away, or do you put it off? When you experience sleepiness at night, do tend to blow it off or get ready for bed? If you are feeling pain in some region of your body—say your foot—do you pay attention, or do you tend to ignore it?

The more you attend to the sensations of your body, the more adept you will be at Intuitive Eating. For example, when you feel your hunger and respond in a timely manner, it makes eating a little easier and more predictable.

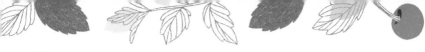

Day
112 **The Upside of Anger**

The upside of anger is that it is a powerful energy that can be harnessed and used to create amazing services, organizations, and actions. On a personal level, it might give you the emotional energy to speak your truth in a relationship—whether it involves people at work, friends, family, or partners. If you grew up in a family in which emotions were silenced, you might minimize or avoid feeling anger. If you grew up in a violent family, witnessing anger can be incredibly scary, and you might find yourself trying to avoid feeling it.

What if you viewed anger as a positive emotion that energizes an action that needs to be taken? How might that change your perspective on feeling angry?

WEEKLY INTENTION

Choose a Fear Food Without Knowing Its Metrics

It wasn't until 1990 that US federal law required nutrition facts on most foods sold in the grocery store. Believe it or not, people used to eat without knowing the exact nutritional information of their food. Today, you can easily find details about what you're eating on most food labels, restaurant menus, phone apps, and the internet.

Consequently, some people manage their food fears by researching the nutritional minutiae of a particular food, such as standard serving size, calories, and macro counts. This includes analyzing a restaurant's web page or searching in an app. The problem with obsessively researching information is that it creates a bigger disconnection between your body and the food you are eating.

This week: Plan to eat a food for which you don't know the nutritional or calorie information. This could be enjoying someone's homemade cookies, eating a dish at a potluck, or choosing a new menu item from a restaurant that you haven't researched.

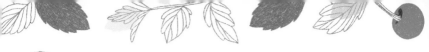
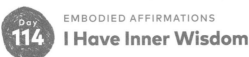

EMBODIED AFFIRMATIONS
Day 114
I Have Inner Wisdom

Diet culture is focused on the external, at the great expense of making you disconnect from and disregard yourself. Powerful inner wisdom exists within you. You were born with it—it just needs to be reawakened.

PRACTICE

Reflect upon a time or situation in which you knew just the right thing to say or do. This could be an action toward yourself or toward another person or animal. Really take your time to recollect. When this situation is clear in your mind, place your awareness on the felt sense of knowing that you have inner wisdom. Now intensify this feeling. (Simply calling it to mind, clearly, and focusing on the feeling is usually enough to amplify the felt sense of the feeling.)

Using this felt knowingness, with your hand on your heart or in a self-hug, slowly repeat three times, *"I have inner wisdom."*

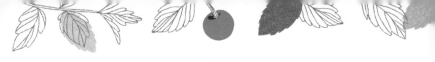

Day
115

INTUITIVE EATING MANTRAS

I am cultivating a healthy
relationship with food,
mind, and body.

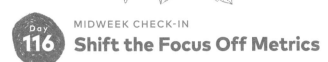

Day 116

MIDWEEK CHECK-IN

Shift the Focus Off Metrics

How are you doing with the weekly intention of choosing a food to eat without knowing its numbers? Letting go of the fixation on external numbers and metrics helps you shift the focus onto what's happening inside your body. It can feel scary and exhilarating at the same time. That's okay. Remember that experiencing fear doesn't mean that you are eating wrong. It just means you are eating differently—with intention and awareness. Over time, you will find fear gradually leaving your plate.

Day 117

MEAL MEDITATIONS

Gift of Hunger

I thank my body for the gift of hunger—
no matter how small or intense.
Hunger communicates the basic human
need to nourish my body.
Hunger is not a symptom to repress.
It's a beautiful cue to attend and befriend.
The presence of hunger adds to the enjoyment of this meal
I'm about to eat.

SELF-CARE

Self-Care for Stressful Times— Your Nonnegotiables

While daily self-care is important, it's especially critical when you are in survival mode from life's curveballs, like getting sick, dealing with a new project deadline, tending to an ill family member, or juggling a variety of unforeseen circumstances. Whom can you ask for help or to whom can you delegate responsibilities? It's helpful to be clear on your nonnegotiables for enduring challenging times. Consider any of the following:

- Getting adequate sleep
- Getting consistent nourishment and meeting your energy needs in a timely manner
- Moving your body as a way to manage stress
- Taking a day off from moving your body, especially when exhausted
- Meditating
- Seeking social support and connection
- Turning down any new projects or responsibilities
- Having spiritual support

LETTING GO OF DIET CULTURE

Embrace Flexibility and Let Go of Rigidity

There's nothing wrong with having preferences around eating, but what's problematic is when they morph into rules and rigidity. As eating becomes narrower and more constricted, overall thought patterns tend to become binary (all or nothing). Your life becomes more and more constrained. What could you do to add flexibility to your eating or movement today?

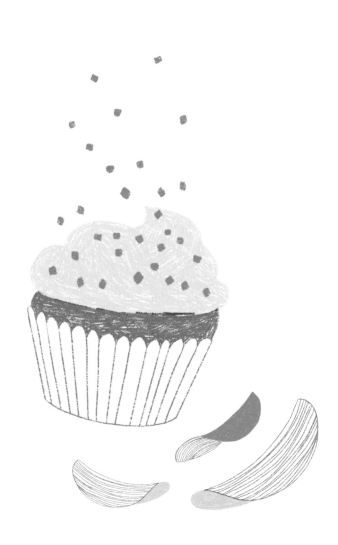

Challenge the Food Police

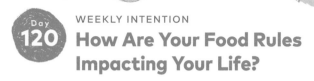

WEEKLY INTENTION

How Are Your Food Rules Impacting Your Life?

You were not born with food rules tattooed on your mouth or stomach. Rather they are a cumulative acquisition that comes from a variety of sources, such as family, friends, community, celebrities, sports figures, coaches, news, media, health professionals, teachers, social media, diet programs, food plans, and research. Fortunately, food rules can be deconstructed and dismantled, which is a key part of regaining your autonomy.

This week: Reflect on your core food rules—the ones that most commonly guide your eating decisions. Where did they come from? (It's okay if you don't know.) How are they serving you, and how do they harm? How do the food rules impact the quality of your life?

SELF-COMPASSION
You Are Not Alone

Most people don't brag about their food or body anxieties. What we hear instead is diet culture's very loud bragging about how easy and effortless it is to shrink the body. (You may have a friend or two who do this, and perhaps you have engaged in this kind of diet talk as well.) It's a form of self-absorption, but most people are unaware of it. When the diet predictably stops working and the euphoria wanes, however, people don't talk about the difficulties they are having with food, body, and mind. It's just not the stuff of party talk or social banter.

The next time you find yourself falling down the rabbit hole of isolation, where you feel like you are the only one having food and body problems, it's important to remember you are not alone.

CULTIVATING TRUST
Keeping Food in the Home

When you feel ready (and have the financial privilege), the act of stocking your pantry and refrigerator is healing. It's a visual reminder of abundance—that you have the food that you need, rejecting the scarcity and fear that diet culture perpetuates. It supports you trusting that you will nourish your body as needed.

Purchasing plenty of previously forbidden foods facilitates the beauty of making peace with foods, which also repairs trust. While it may be impossible to imagine, the foods that used to haunt and call out your name will no longer hold power over you.

MIDWEEK CHECK-IN
Inner Food Rules

Food rules are a cage that binds and restricts your freedom to eat. Cultivating nonjudgmental *awareness* of these rules is a key step toward liberation. It's a stance of gentle observation of your thoughts without condemning or judging them. After all, you can't deconstruct or uproot what you are not aware of. What have you noticed so far?

Day
124

INTUITIVE EATING MANTRAS

All bodies are worthy
of dignity and respect,
including my own.

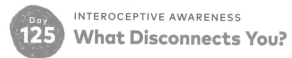

Day 125

What Disconnects You?

It's helpful to know your vulnerability points—situations or activities that may disconnect you from the felt senses in your body. These can range from fun activities that pull you away from all sense of time to sheer stress and exhaustion where you are simultaneously feeling wired and tired.

Which of the following might be your vulnerability spots, where you unintentionally disconnect from your body?

- Watching a movie

- Reading a page-turner

- Scrolling through endless social media feeds

- Channel surfing television shows, not ever really settling on one

- Working on an exciting project

- Using substances to escape, such as alcohol or cannabis

What would you add to this list that matches your tendencies and vulnerability?

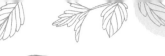

BODY APPRECIATION
Connection in Relationships

Day 126

Your dear body is capable of so many things, including connecting with others. Humans are wired to connect—and touching is one way we do so. Consider the impact this has on your relationships. Think about how having a body—your body—allows you to make contact with others, such as a giving a reassuring hug to a loved one, holding your child's hand, kissing a lover, or giving a colleague a high five for a job well done.

Reflect on how *your* body allows you to bond with others. What types of physical connection are the most meaningful to you?

Body Gratitude: Thank you, body, for allowing me to grow closer to others by _____.
(State your favorite way to connect with your body.)

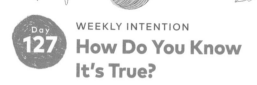

WEEKLY INTENTION
How Do You Know It's True?

Repeating the same thought or rule over and over again can make it feel like a fact. After a while, these thoughts and rules may evolve into an absolute belief system. For some people, this system is almost like a religion, complete with evangelists espousing their dietary tenets.

The problem is that rigid food rules impact your quality of life and relationships by adding unnecessary stress and anxiety. Sometimes it's easier to let go of rules when you can see the futility or the lack of evidence for them. More importantly, you see that the rules impede where you want to go, toward food freedom.

This week: Explore your top food rules. Are they true? Who says so—what is the source? What is the context? Does the rule help me become freer and more flexible with my eating? Does it support my relationships and things that matter to me? What would happen if I was more flexible with this rule? What would happen if I stopped following it altogether?

Day 128

I Am Resilient, There Isn't Anything I Can't Handle

Diet culture can leave you doubting yourself and feeling like a failure because diet after diet hasn't "worked." Remember, it's the dieting and food plans that have failed you. Your abilities as a person have absolutely nothing to do with your abilities in diet culture.

PRACTICE

Reflect upon a time in which you handled a difficult situation with resiliency. When this occasion is clear in your mind, place your awareness on the felt sense of knowing that you have resiliency. Now intensify this feeling. (Simply calling it to mind, clearly, and focusing on the feeling is usually enough to amplify the felt sense of the feeling.)

Using this felt knowingness, slowly repeat three times, *"I am resilient; there isn't anything I can't handle."*

LOVING BOUNDARIES

Little Self-Boundaries—Not Automatically Responding

Here are some very simple actions that you can take that will give you breathing room and won't interrupt your workflow or train of thought: Try *not* to automatically

- Reply to a text, rather respond at your convenience;

- Answer your phone, especially when it's not a good time for you to talk;

- Participate in conversations that drain your energy;

- Reply to emails, instead prioritizing when and how you will respond.

MIDWEEK CHECK-IN

Inner Food Police

The inner food police is the internalized voice of diet culture. The rules generated by the food police can feel like absolute facts, because they've been repeated so many times. They are chanted and reinforced from nearly every corner of society from social media to headline news. It can feel difficult to uproot them, but fear not, it's workable. What have you noticed so far?

Day
131

INTUITIVE EATING MANTRAS

Intuitive Eating is an intimate journey of coming back to my personal home.

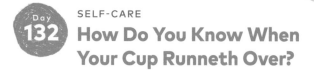

Day 132 How Do You Know When Your Cup Runneth Over?

It's important to recognize when you are getting pulled in too many directions. It's not very hard to recognize the impact when this affects activities and obligations that you barely tolerate. But what about when you are doing too many things that involve your passions? The effects can be just as detrimental. Here are some signs you could be doing too much:

- There's a change in your moods.

- You have difficulty falling asleep or are waking up too early.

- You have increased anxious thoughts.

- You are more impatient and irritable.

- You feel as if you'll never be able to catch up.

- You have less time for friends.

- You stay up late and don't get enough sleep.

- You have increased stress.

REFLECT
When you find yourself in these situations, what could you let go of or delay? Is it possible to build in more breaks between projects and activities? What if you valued downtime just as much as time engaged in activities that you love? How might this affect the quality of your life?

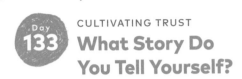

CULTIVATING TRUST

Day 133

What Story Do You Tell Yourself?

Our minds are natural storytellers. They try to make sense of our place in the world and keep us safe. The problem is that these stories are just that—stories, not facts. Even so, these narratives influence your reality, especially if you internalize them as truth. The stories you tell yourself about your body have a big impact on self-trust. What are some of the body stories that you tell yourself? Do these move you closer to or further away from self-connection?

The good news is that you can change and release the narratives that no longer serve you, but first you need to be aware of the story line. Reflect on how it would feel to adopt one (or more!) of the following as a pillar of your inner dialogue:

- My body has kept me alive, whether I trust my body or not.

- My body is the house of my spirit, my soul, and my wisdom.

- My body is worthy of being treated with dignity and respect.

- My body deserves nourishment, each and every day.

- My body has healed my physical wounds, whether I love it or not.

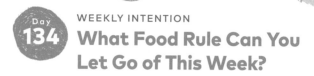

WEEKLY INTENTION

What Food Rule Can You Let Go of This Week?

Food rules accumulate like scratches and dents on luggage—you are not sure how they got there, but, over time, they can wear you down. Challenging the food police is about identifying and letting go of rigid food rules that dictate how, when, and what you eat—regardless of how your body is feeling or what food sounds satisfying and delicious.

You have already reflected on how food rules affect the quality of your life. The problematic rules tend to be inflexible, make you feel guilty or anxious, or impact your ability to socialize and eat out with other people. The rules tend to be rooted with the words *should* and *shouldn't*.

This week: What would you need in order to let go of one food rule? For some people, it's accepting the initial fear that comes with change. Each time you increase flexibility with your eating, you are one step closer to freedom. What food rule are you willing to let go of this week?

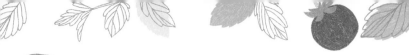

Day 135

LETTING GO OF DIET CULTURE
Let Go of Fear-Based Eating

Adding fear and guilt to a meal is one of the fastest ways to rob the joy and pleasure from eating. The presence of these emotions is understandable with the proliferation of sensational, fearmongering documentaries and headline news that demand attention and make for enticing clickbait. The media seldom delves into, let alone acknowledges, the complexity and nuances of nutrition science. Instead, cherry-picked statistics and studies tend to overshadow balanced counterpoints. In truth, rarely are there absolutes with eating.

Here are three questions to ask when evaluating food claims:

1. *Is that really true, and how do you know?*

2. *Who says, and what is the source?*

3. *What is the counterpoint?*

One day, meal, or snack will not make or break your health. What fear do you need to release to bring pleasure and peace back to your plate?

PRINCIPLE 4. CHALLENGE THE FOOD POLICE   141

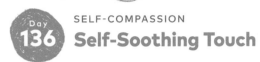

SELF-COMPASSION

Self-Soothing Touch

Touch is an incredibly powerful way to help you self-soothe. The simple act of touch activates part of the nervous system (the parasympathetic system), which helps you feel safe and calms distressing emotions. Parents instinctively trigger this reaction when they pick up a crying baby and rock the little one in their arms.

There's also another biological bonus of touch: It releases the "cuddle" hormone, oxytocin, which plays a role in social bonding and reducing stress.[13] Here are some ways to explore self-soothing touch:

- *Run* your fingers throughout your scalp.
- *Place* your hand on your heart.
- *Rub* the back of your head, where your skull meets your neck.
- *Give* your shoulder a light rub with your opposite hand.

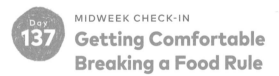

Day 137

MIDWEEK CHECK-IN

Getting Comfortable Breaking a Food Rule

Once you decide that a rule is no longer serving you and that you are ready to let go, there's nothing to break. In the beginning, it can feel as if you are doing something wrong. The uneasiness just indicates that it's an unfamiliar behavior—you are in new territory. New ways of being and behaving sometimes feel uncomfortable or awkward, but that does not mean the change is bad or wrong. It's just different.

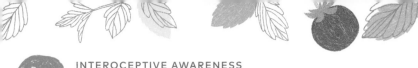

Day 138

INTEROCEPTIVE AWARENESS

Befriending Your Body as a Valued Messenger

What if you viewed your body as a kind friend, a messenger with powerful information to help get your needs met? What would you need in order to attend to and befriend your body and hear its messages? Perhaps it means taking a few pauses through-out the day and simply listening to the felt sense—the physical sensations that your body is offering. What if you valued these messages, rather than turn away or disregard them? How might that affect your quality of life?

Day 139

INTUITIVE EATING MANTRAS

Shame has no place in Intuitive Eating.

Day 140

MEAL MEDITATIONS

Eating Without Guilt or Moral Dilemma

May I uncouple morality from my eating.
May I disengage my identity from what I eat.
May I recognize that virtue is not attained by the foods I choose to eat.
May I appreciate that my food choices do not reflect my character.

Day 141

WEEKLY INTENTION

Using Guilt as a Gateway to Healing

The sensation of guilt does not feel good in the body. So when it arises, you are usually well aware of its presence. This offers a valuable opportunity to get curious and shine the light of awareness to illuminate an unspoken food rule or belief.

This week: Notice when a sensation of guilt arises—where do you feel it in your body?

Contemplate the following prompts:

- *What belief or rule might be triggering this feeling?*

- *Does this rule help me stay present and connected to my body, or does it disrupt self-connection? Do I value this belief or rule?*

- *What do I need in order to let go of this guilt-inducing belief or rule?*

Day 142

I Am Not My Thoughts

Thoughts are powerful. Yet they are nothing more than the narrative of your mind—your inner storyteller of perceptions. Thoughts are not facts, and they certainly don't define you! It's all too easy to get wrapped up in your thoughts and to over-identify with them, because in the moment, thoughts often *feel* true. It's especially problematic when you are having shaming or mean thoughts about yourself.

PRACTICE

Reflect upon a time or situation in which you realized that a thought pattern was not true. Perhaps it was during a difficult time in your life that felt fixed and permanent. When the situation is clear in your mind, place your awareness on the felt sense of knowing that you are not your body, and you are not your thought patterns. Now intensify this feeling. (Simply calling it to mind, clearly, and focusing on the feeling is usually enough to amplify the felt sense of the feeling.)

Using this felt knowingness, with your hand on your heart or in a self-hug, slowly repeat three times, *"I am not my thoughts."*

EMOTIONS AND CRAVINGS

Day 143

Drop the Story Line

Emotions reside in our bodies. Rather than paying attention to the physical felt sense of the emotion, our mind is quick to make up a story that *feels* true. It is the narrative of the mind, our clever internal story maker, that prolongs emotional sensation. It's the added gasoline to the fire. The next time you experience an emotion, try dropping the narrative. Instead, shift your awareness into your body. Notice the physical sensation of emotion—where do you feel it in your body? Get curious and notice how long the sensation lasts. Every time you get pulled back in the story line (your thoughts), kindly redirect your mind to the sensations in your body.

MIDWEEK CHECK-IN

Day 144

The Benefit of Noticing Guilt

There is a paradox of noticing the unpleasant sensation of guilt from eating: You discover a food rule or belief that's holding you back from experiencing true freedom with eating and the pleasure that comes with it. When you identify the rule at the root of food guilt, you are better equipped to challenge it. Over time, as you practice rejecting or talking back to the rule or belief, guilt will dissipate.

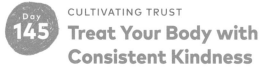

Day 145

CULTIVATING TRUST

Treat Your Body with Consistent Kindness

Have you ever seen how a mistreated puppy or dog behaves? It's wary, and may snarl and bite if you attempt to pet it. These are protective self-defense mechanisms. The puppy doesn't trust you because it has been mistreated. These behaviors are understandable but not endearing, which may cause you to dislike the puppy.

Your body is like that puppy. It suffers at the hand of culturally sanctioned fat phobia, the roots of which have been traced back to the seventeenth century and the origins of racism, patriarchy, and religious dogma.[14]

Healing your relationship with your body is about treating it with dignity and respect, meeting its needs regardless of how you feel about it. In other words, you don't have to like your body to cultivate the practice of trust, kindness, and respect. Over time, you will be able to appreciate the miraculous ways in which your body functions and shows up for you day after day.

BODY APPRECIATION

Cultivate and Lean In to Your Character Strengths

Researchers from the field of positive psychology have identified twenty-four core character strengths that are outlined in the following list. We all possess strengths, but they are expressed and valued differently for each person. Research shows that cultivating these strengths contributes to a fulfilling life, improved well-being, and flourishing.[15] Imagine shifting your time and energy to cultivating your character strengths, rather than denigrating or changing your body.

View the chart that follows; with which of these strengths do you most identify? (To learn more about character strengths and take a free validated assessment, see Viacharacter.org/character-strengths.)

In order to lean in to your character strengths, begin by reminding yourself that you are more than a body. Next, shift your focus to the top one or two character strengths that you appreciate about yourself. Your statement might sound like this:

I am more than a body and I appreciate my _____.

Creativity	Spirituality	Modesty
Curiosity	Bravery	Prudence
Open-Mindedness	Persistence	Self-Regulation
Love of Learning	Zest	Appreciation
Perspective-Taking	Fairness	Gratitude
Authenticity	Leadership	Kindness
Hope	Teamwork	Love
Humor	Forgiveness	Social Intelligence

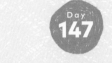

Day
147

INTUITIVE EATING MANTRAS

Through Intuitive Eating,
I am honoring my unique
needs with kindness.

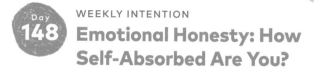

WEEKLY INTENTION

Emotional Honesty: How Self-Absorbed Are You?

The more you are steeped in diet culture and food rules, the more self-absorbed you tend to become about what you can and cannot eat. It's a mental hijacking that is revealed via diet talk in many social settings. And most folks are not confronted about their verbal "health" obsession. Frankly, people just don't know what to say to them. Adding fuel to the fire, diet culture behaviors are often praised.

This week: Explore the impact of diet culture as your object of attention, with kind, nonjudgmental awareness:

- Do you often talk a lot about your newest food plan or diet, or why you aren't eating a particular food? Does this happen in most settings in which there is food?

- Do you usually initiate these conversations?

- Do you look for opportunities to talk about your latest food regimen?

- How often is this part of your small talk with strangers?

- Do you find that you are trying to talk people into your way of eating?

- Do you verbally judge or shame people about their food choices?

Answering yes to most of these questions? Please don't be harsh on yourself. It's a sign of diet culture's powerful grasp, and might also be an indicator that you are not eating enough food.

Consider other things you could talk about other than your eating—you'll make deeper, more authentic connections with people.

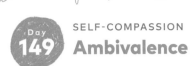

Day 149

SELF-COMPASSION
Ambivalence

You might want both peace with your body and food AND a smaller body. This doesn't make you a bad person. It's normal to feel ambivalent and conflicted when you've had a lifetime pursuit and mindset of wanting to change your body. You are the byproduct of diet culture, which now sadly even infiltrates a lot of health care. You (and most of our culture) have been conditioned with the thin ideal, which also serves as a form of virtue signaling.

The challenge is that pursuing a smaller body size interferes with the process of Intuitive Eating, and it reinforces fat phobia. The real path toward freedom and peace begins when you can truly let go. This allows you to tune in to your body's needs, breaking free from external rules and distractions. It's okay if you don't feel ready. As a baby step, can you put the idea of weight on the back burner? This acknowledges that the desire is there, but you are not acting on it.

It's also normal to harbor fantasies of a smaller body even while you are truly on the path of Intuitive Eating. This journey is not about perfection; rather, it's about unlearning and letting go of the attachment to body size. This takes time.

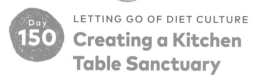

Day 150
Creating a Kitchen Table Sanctuary

Eating is meant to be pleasurable. Demonizing foods takes away the joy of eating and undermines our connections with both others and ourselves at mealtime. Our homes and our kitchen tables are our sacred places. We can stop the legacy of diet culture by creating our own sanctuary for nourishing our bodies by adding guidelines to the table. Regardless of where you eat in your home,[16] consider including the following:

- We nourish our bodies, regardless of size or shape.

- We appreciate the food we are able to eat.

- We do not criticize how much or what anyone is eating, including ourselves.

- We don't talk about diets and the people following them.

What else would you add?

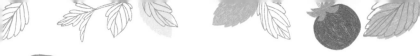

Day 151 MIDWEEK CHECK-IN

Impact of Self-Absorption

This week you've been noticing your possible self-absorption with eating. How have you been doing with that? This may feel especially hard because it's really about the impact of your self-absorption on other people. And that can be really challenging and painful to own. That's why kindness and gentleness toward yourself is crucial. An especially brave step could be to ask a couple of inner-circle friends, whom you trust, who also seem to have a peaceful relationship with their eating and their body, "Do you think I talk a lot about my eating and/or body?"

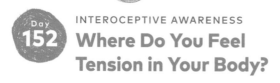

INTEROCEPTIVE AWARENESS
Where Do You Feel Tension in Your Body?

Stress, in its subtler forms, can be experienced as tension. How often might you be navigating daily life with tension in places such as your jaw, neck, shoulders, head, eyes, upper or lower back, or stomach?

PRACTICE

You can do this practice seated, standing, or lying down if you wish. Get in a comfortable position of your choosing. Then take a couple of relaxing breaths. Place one hand on an area of your body where you are likely to feel tension, perhaps your neck. From *inside* your body, notice what sensation you feel. What word would describe this sensation (see list on page 65)? Does it have a shape? Does it have a temperature? Does it have a color? Does it have a texture?

There's no right or wrong way to perceive sensations. Just notice it, without trying to change or fix anything. As you give sustained attention to this sensation, what happens? Does it stay the same? If it changes, what sensation word would describe it?

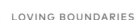

Day 153

Five More Ways to Say No

- Thank you for thinking of me, but I'm not available.

- Unfortunately, I'm not able to _____.

- I'm not comfortable with _____.

- I'm not able to add another project.

- No, it doesn't work for me.

Day 154

INTUITIVE EATING MANTRAS

I listen and respond
to the needs
of my body in
a timely manner.

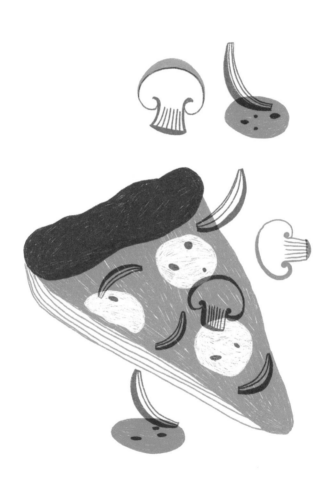

Satisfaction Factor

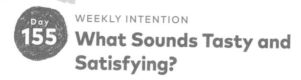

WEEKLY INTENTION

What Sounds Tasty and Satisfying?

Day 155

Part of cultivating satisfaction in your eating is figuring out what sounds satisfying to eat. While this might sound incredibly easy at first glance, it can be a daunting task. When you've chronically abdicated your eating choices to some external food plan or guru, it's common to lose sight of yourself, your needs, and your preferences.

Sometimes, simply asking yourself what sounds satisfying to eat will point you in the right direction. It's okay if you don't know—it's really a common challenge in the beginning when you've been eating based on rules. Every eating experience is an opportunity to learn more about yourself. Only you know what will ultimately satisfy and sustain you.

This week. When choosing a meal or snack, ask yourself what sounds satisfying. Consider these factors to help get clarity using this question: Do I want something _____?

- Spicy or bland
- Hot or cold
- Sweet or sour
- Crunchy or smooth
- Hearty or light
- Liquid, like soup, or chewy, like a sandwich

CULTIVATING TRUST

There Is No Failure, Just Discovery and Learning

It's important to remember that Intuitive Eating is a journey of self-discovery and learning; there is no failure. Diet culture instills a binary way of thinking—pass or fail, good or bad, on my food plan or off my food plan. This type of thinking can lead you to lose trust in yourself after your perceived food mistakes. Eventually, it starts to creep into other areas of your life and erode self-trust even further.

To develop a shift in perspectives, operate from the framework of learning, rather than a binary pass or fail. During (or after) difficult times, try asking yourself: What can I learn from this situation? What might I do differently if I find myself in similar circumstances? Focusing on learning helps you let go. It also gives meaning to something otherwise viewed as a negative. More importantly, it honors your ability to learn and grow, which nurtures confidence and self-trust.

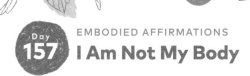

EMBODIED AFFIRMATIONS

Day 157

I Am Not My Body

Diet culture objectifies bodies, which can easily condition you to believe that's all you are. This is a huge disservice to your humanity—you are so much more than a body. Consider the celebrated humanitarians like Mother Theresa or Nelson Mandela—their actions are what made them great, not the size or shape of their bodies. You have a body, but your identity is not your body.

PRACTICE

Reflect upon a time or situation in which you realized that you are more than a body. This could be a time when you were moved spiritually, poetically, creatively, or relationally. When this situation is clear in your mind, place your awareness on the felt sense of knowing that your worth is not tied up in your body, that you are more than a body. Now intensify this feeling. (Simply calling it to mind, clearly, and focusing on the feeling is usually enough to amplify the felt sense of the feeling.)

Using this felt knowingness, with your hand on your heart or in a self-hug, slowly repeat three times, *"I am not my body."*

MIDWEEK CHECK-IN

Connection with the Pleasure of What Sounds Good

What have you discovered so far about connecting with the sensory pleasures of taste and satisfaction? Did anything surprise you? It's not unusual to fear the experience of enjoyment with eating, in part because diet culture perpetuates the idea that enjoying food is shameful, dangerous, and wrong. Another contributing factor to this fear is puritanical religious roots, upon which many societies were founded or colonized. Rediscovering your inner body wisdom through Intuitive Eating involves a lot of deconditioning and unlearning. This process takes time, but know that healing your relationship with food, body, and mind is possible.

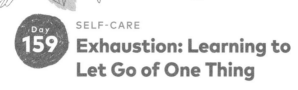

SELF-CARE

Exhaustion: Learning to Let Go of One Thing

Feeling drained and depleted sets you up for vulnerability that's driven by exhaustion. Your thinking gets foggy, and it's easier to become hijacked by emotions. Everything just seems more exhausting and effortful. Just the idea of pushing a microwave button sounds too exhausting, as does tearing the lid off a yogurt container.

In these times, it's incredibly helpful to have a contingency plan in place—or to start cultivating one. What's one thing you can let go of during these trying times? Maybe it's taking the night off from cooking. Perhaps it's going to bed an hour earlier. Possibly, it's letting the laundry pile up. Or maybe, it's rescheduling a meeting or opting out of a social gathering.

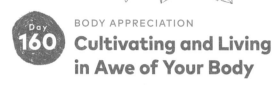

BODY APPRECIATION

Cultivating and Living in Awe of Your Body

Every cell in your body works around the clock just to keep you alive. Upon reflection, it's rather extraordinary. Yet we often take it for granted. Imagine if you lived in awe of what your body does for you each and every day.

Awe is a complex emotion that imparts self-transcendence, shifting our focus away from ourselves and helping us feel more connected to part of a larger whole.[17] In this way, body awe can help you shift your attention away from your appearance.

What might you be in awe of body-wise? Perhaps that your body can heal itself? Without your conscious control, each beat of your heart pumps red blood cells to deliver vital oxygen to your lungs. Your immune system silently fights infections without you lifting a finger.

When you factor in that your body is also the house of your values, character strengths, and humanity—and the place where life happens: connection to other people, creativity, emotions, cognitions, and pleasure—it's rather incredible. But when our culture objectifies our body, it erases and devalues all of this magic—the miracle of life and connection.

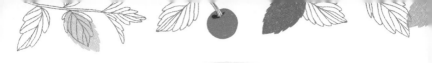

Day
161

INTUITIVE EATING MANTRAS

Nourishing your body is a life-affirming act.

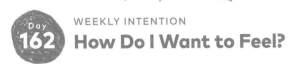

How Do I Want to Feel?

Satisfaction from eating includes feeling content and sustained after you have eaten. That's why, ultimately, neither under- nor overeating is satisfying. The practice of Intuitive Eating integrates the wisdom of both body and mind.

This week: As you are contemplating what you would like to eat this week, consider how you would like to feel when you are finished eating.

- *Do you want to feel sustained for a long period of time?* Perhaps you are preparing to take a long flight, sit in school for an extended period of time, or work long hours before you have another opportunity to eat. In these types of situations, it may be useful to eat a meal that sustains you. Consider your own history of eating; what types of foods or meals keep you sustained for longer periods of time?

- *Do you want to feel content, yet not in digestive overload?* Consider situations like when you are speaking in public or going to participate in an activity such as yoga or a dance class. Considering your past eating experiences, what types of foods or meals keep you energized without bogging you down?

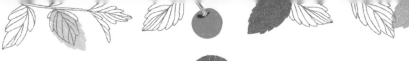

Day
163

MEAL MEDITATIONS

Awakened Eating

May my eyes enjoy the colors on my plate.
May my tongue experience the nuances of flavor.
May my nose delight in the complexities of aroma.
May my ears appreciate the sounds of dining.
May my mind be free of the eating entanglements of judgment.

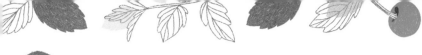

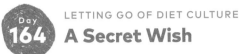

LETTING GO OF DIET CULTURE
A Secret Wish

Though you may have intellectually rejected diet culture, you might still feel a longing, a secret wish, for a different body. This is especially true for folks in marginalized or larger bodies who don't align with the narrow cultural ideals of beauty and worth.

You might have experienced living in a smaller body for a period of time, which makes diet culture's claims especially seductive. The truth is restricting food in that way is just not sustainable. That's because at the biological level, your cells are clinging on for dear life and trying to survive by doing things like slowing down your metabolism and ramping up your desire for food.

Rather than hold on to hopes and fantasies, reflect on the ways in which your life could be fuller, more engaged, and more enjoyable in your here-and-now body. It's okay to feel sad; that's a normal part of letting go. Underneath that sadness, you might find anger toward a society that unfairly places our bodies in a hierarchy of size.

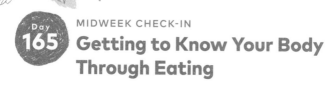

MIDWEEK CHECK-IN

Getting to Know Your Body Through Eating

Dieting is a form of disembodiment—with each diet or food plan, you become more and more disconnected from your body's signals and needs. In the beginning of your Intuitive Eating journey, it can feel really hard to consider how you want to feel when you finish a meal or snack. Or, you might know how you want to feel, but you have no idea what types of meals or snacks will get you there. That's okay. In time, and with patience and awareness, you will truly know from your own experience. Every time you eat is an opportunity to learn more about yourself and your body.

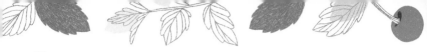

Day 166

How Does the Process of Eating Feel?

Choose a meal or snack today where you can focus on the varied sensations of eating. Upon taking your first bit of food, notice

- *The texture of the food while you are chewing.* Does the consistency change markedly (like chewing a bite of a sandwich) or is it a subtle shift (like when eating a spoonful of yogurt)? Just notice.

- *The sensation of swallowing.* How does it feel? How often do you take this bodily act of eating for granted?

- *The swallowed food as it travels down your esophagus.* Place your awareness on this feeling. Get curious. How far down can you track this sensation?

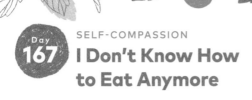

Day 167

I Don't Know How to Eat Anymore

This is a common and exasperating belief after following food, wellness, and lifestyle plans (a.k.a. forms of dieting). It's incredibly frustrating to feel confident and successful in other parts of your life, but not with eating. You may know macros, points, or calories in foods—like a computer database. But this information isn't self-knowledge and doesn't facilitate true self-connection with your mind and body. These metrics are external information that have little to do with your unique and specific needs.

It's really understandable if you feel as if you don't know how to eat anymore. You likely have been living in diet culture for months, years, or even decades. You are not alone. Teaching yourself how to eat again is a matter of learning to listen deeply and respond in a timely manner to the needs of your body. This takes time and practice.

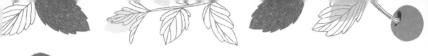

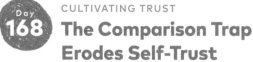

CULTIVATING TRUST

Day 168

The Comparison Trap Erodes Self-Trust

No human body has identical needs; we all have different genetics, activity levels, gut microbiomes, life experiences, and conditions. Even so, it's common for people to compare their eating to that of others, including complete strangers! Comparative eating weakens self-connection and erodes trust. (It would be like trying to compare the amount you pee to someone else! Sounds ridiculous, right? But for some reason, when it comes to eating, it is a socially normative practice.)

If you find yourself in the food comparison trap, shift your attention back to your body, and kindly ask yourself: *What do I need, what sounds good, and what will satisfy me?* The more you ask (and answer) those questions, the more you build connection and trust with yourself.

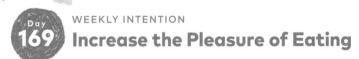

WEEKLY INTENTION
Increase the Pleasure of Eating

The pleasurable aspects of eating can be missed if you're in the habit of eating while distracted, because the mind can only place its awareness on one thing at time. Just like a camera lens, it will only see (and experience) what it focuses on. You miss out on the full experience of eating when you are multitasking, such as while watching TV, scrolling through social media, reading, or paying bills. This can leave you feeling less satisfied.

This Week. Choose to eat one meal or snack a day without engaging in another activity. Notice how it feels to eat without distraction. Is the process of eating more enjoyable? Does the food taste more satisfying? Is it easier to identify emerging fullness?

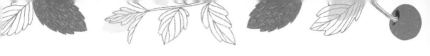

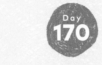

Day
170

INTUITIVE EATING MANTRAS

Intuitive Eating is about cultivating a healthy relationship with myself—not the pursuit of weight loss.

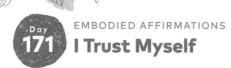

Day 171
I Trust Myself

Abiding by diet culture's rules and expectations erodes self-trust, which subsequently spills into other areas of your life. It's important to affirm that you can trust yourself.

> **PRACTICE**
> Recall a time in which you truly trusted yourself; perhaps it's a difficult situation in which you made a good decision or a time when you sensed something was off and trusted yourself to leave and get out of harm's way.
>
> Now, intensify this feeling of trusting knowingness, and with your hand on your heart or in a self-hug, slowly repeat three times, "*I trust myself.*"

MIDWEEK CHECK-IN

Day 172
Letting Go of Multitasking to Increase Satisfaction and Connection

Though eating without distraction may sound straightforward, it can be challenging if you are accustomed to eating while multitasking. In the beginning there can be reluctance to taking this step. That's completely understandable. Try not to judge yourself for feeling reluctant. Ease into this by trying to eat without distraction for just part of the meal—say the first five or ten minutes.

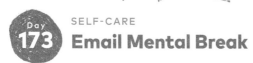

SELF-CARE

Email Mental Break

Receiving emails is like an unrelenting waterfall—it never stops. It can feel like Whac-A-Mole: As soon as you answer one email, another one pops up demanding your attention. Sometimes, you just need a break.

What if you set up an automatic away message for your email to give yourself a mental break? (Most people do this when they go on vacation, but you can use this setting at any time.) It manages expectations for when you'll reply to a person's email.

Perhaps an away message could look like this:

"I'm away from the internet and will not be checking or responding to emails until my return on (insert date or time)."

LOVING BOUNDARIES

Boundaries about Diet Talk— Conversation Shifters

It's helpful to have some automatic responses to change the subject when people start talking about their latest diet or lifestyle change. See which response resonates best with you:

- "Can we change the topic to something other than bodies and diets? I'd love to hear about your _____ (last vacation, book you just finished, favorite movie)."

- "Dieting has been harmful to me; I'm trying to steer clear of these conversations, and would love it if could we talk about something else."

- "I'm trying to focus on connecting with my body, and these conversations leave me feeling confused and doubting myself. I'd appreciate if we could talk about a different topic."

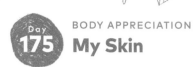

Day 175

My Skin

Your one and only body works hard to do extraordinary things, which is often taken for granted. Consider your skin—the largest *organ* of your body. With a lifespan of just about four weeks, your skin cells fall off and die, and your body sheds about 50 million cells each day. In other words, your skin is in a constant state of regeneration.[18]

Your skin also plays many roles in keeping you healthy, including regulating your body temperature and providing a protective barrier against germs and toxic substances. It's integral to healing too. When you get a cut or scrape or skin infection, your body makes new skin cells to replace the skin you have lost.

Body Gratitude: I appreciate my skin, which helps keep me healthy.

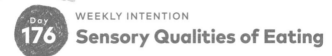

Day 176
Sensory Qualities of Eating

Placing your awareness on the sensory qualities of eating cultivates greater satisfaction and pleasure with your meals and snacks. It's all too easy to bring our hectic, rushed mentality to the table, which distracts us from the here-and-now sensual qualities of eating.

This Week: Choose one daily meal or snack on which to place your focused attention. This will be a two-step practice followed by a reflection:

First, notice the overall aroma and display of food in front of you. Second, get curious and place your awareness on these sensory qualities. With each bite of food, notice the

- *Sight* of food on your fork or spoon in your hand;
- *Sound* of food as you unwrap it, bite into it, or slurp it;
- *Smell* of food just before biting into it;
- *Touch* of food as it passes your lips onto your tongue and into your mouth;
- *Taste* each bite of food, observing the nuances and notes of flavor as you chew.

REFLECT
Did anything surprise you with this practice? Perhaps you found it easier to eat without distraction because the mind had something specific to observe?

LETTING GO OF DIET CULTURE

Getting Rid of the Mental Load from Diet Culture

There is often a perpetual background of anxiety that occupies your mind when you are consumed with body-loathing and following food rules. When diet culture's mental clutter is cleared away, you can be more present in your relationships, which is a gift to both yourself and the important people in your life. You are able to move through the world with more ease, flexibility, and peace. How has your mind freed up some space since letting go of diet culture?

Day
178

INTUITIVE EATING MANTRAS

In order for me to make peace with food, I need to stop the war with my body.

Day 179

Connecting with Your Senses Increases Satisfaction: Sight, Sound, Smell, Touch, and Taste

What is your favorite sensory experience of eating? Consider making that the focal point while you eat. It's also common to be delighted with different sensory experiences from different foods—such as the fragrant aroma of baked cookies or the sight of a colorful salad on your plate. There is no wrong way to savor your senses with eating.

CULTIVATING TRUST

Letting Go of the Body as a Scapegoat

Part of being a human is experiencing a wide range of emotions. Generally, feelings such as anger, grief, stress, and anxiety have a felt sense of physical unpleasantness. You may feel heavy with sadness or feel the burdensome weight on your shoulders with unrelenting stress.

When you have been at war with your body, negative emotions tend to get entangled with your physical self. Because your body is the physical holder of emotions, it easily gets blamed and becomes the scapegoat for life's challenges. Over time, with the unrelenting barbs from diet culture and perpetual self-loathing, it's easy to latch onto the idea that changing your body will change your life.

If you find yourself in an emotionally loaded situation and are feeling the urge to fixate on shrinking your body, come home to your body by shifting your awareness to the inside. Pause and kindly ask yourself, *What am I feeling emotionally, right now? What might I need?*

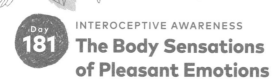

Day 181
The Body Sensations of Pleasant Emotions

It's easy to get caught up in the vortex of negative emotions and the accompanying physical sensations—like the gut-wrenching emptiness of a romantic breakup. But how often do we really get curious and swept up in the physical sensations of joyful and contented times?

PRACTICE

Today, when you notice a moment of happiness, joy, or content-ment, lean in and pay attention to how it *feels* in your body. Perhaps there is a lightness, an openness, or a relaxed radiating sensation? How would you describe the physical sensation? (See list on page 65.)

SELF-COMPASSION

Day 182
Unconditional Self-Love

Body shame is socially conditioned. You were not born hating your body, but you live in a culture that denigrates bodies and taught you to do the same. Loathing your body seeps into how you feel about your overall self. It's hard to take care of something that you hate, including your sense of self and your body.

REFLECT
If you loved yourself unconditionally, how would you talk to yourself today? If that idea seems like too far of a stretch, think about how you would talk to a friend to whom you extend unconditional regard and dignity.

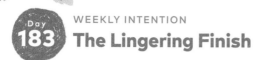

A delightful component of eating is discovering the lingering taste in your mouth after you have swallowed your food. In wine tasting, this is known as the "finish." Experiencing the aftertaste contributes to your satisfaction in eating. But it's subtle and can be easily missed if you tend to eat fast or while distracted.

This week: After you swallow a bite of food, pause. Place your attention on the aftertaste. In the beginning, it may feel easier to notice the aftertaste by lightly rolling your tongue along your upper and lower teeth. In time, just your awareness alone will be enough to make you savor this experience.

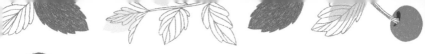

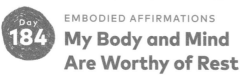

EMBODIED AFFIRMATIONS

Day **184**

My Body and Mind Are Worthy of Rest

We live in a culture that values "the grind," where rest is often not valued. Diet culture reinforces this by disconnecting you from your body, often to the point of feeling numb, which inhibits you from noticing when your body needs a break. In order to thrive and feel at our best, we need rest.

PRACTICE

Reflect on a time when you really allowed yourself to relax and rest. How did that affect your energy levels and mental outlook?

Using this feeling, with your hand on your heart or in a self-hug, slowly repeat three times, *"My body and mind are worthy of rest."*

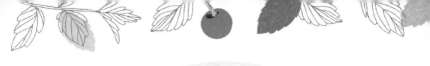

INTUITIVE EATING MANTRAS

Intuitive Eating is
an inside job that lets
me connect to my
body sensations.

MIDWEEK CHECK-IN
The Joy of the Aftertaste

Day 186

Simply noticing the aftertaste extends the joy of eating. It's a nuance of the pleasure of eating that's easily missed if you are not paying attention. If you find yourself rushing through life and your to-do list, for instance, that hectic mentality easily spills over into the eating process. Some people put food in their mouths before even swallowing the previous bite. What have you discovered about the aftertaste?

Day 187

MEAL MEDITATIONS
May I Be Willing

May I be willing to eat without distraction.
May I be willing to connect with my body.
May I be willing to cultivate awareness.
May I be willing to try new eating experiences.

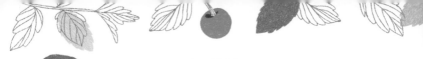

EMOTIONS AND CRAVINGS

Day 188

Three Gratitudes

Sometimes, we need a broader perspective when we are experiencing uncomfortable emotions. Try this technique the next time you feel an unpleasant feeling.

Label or describe your unpleasant emotion (own it, don't dismiss or minimize it).

AND . . .

Describe three things you are grateful for, even while you are feeling an uncomfortable emotion.

So the practice sounds like this:

I am feeling _____,

AND I am grateful for these three things in my life:

1. _____ ,

2. _____ ,

3. _____ .

Example: I am feeling sad, AND I am grateful for my freedom, my ability to care for a dog, and my flexible work schedule.

Day 189

Why Body Compliments Are Harmful

Diet culture focuses on appearance, and it's really common to give compliments based on how someone looks, especially around body weight. While they may come from good intentions, body-based comments have a negative impact by perpetuating weight stigma. Regardless of your intention, commenting on a person's weight is problematic for many reasons:

- You might be complimenting someone's eating disorder. (You cannot tell by the look of a person if they have been engaging in eating disorder behaviors, such as purging, restricting, or using laxatives.)

- The person might have cancer or some disease that they don't want to discuss.

- The person may be going through a stressful time, such as marital strife, mental illness, or depression.

- It objectifies a person and reinforces weight stigma.

- It reinforces a hierarchy of body sizes.

- It suggests that they did not look good before.

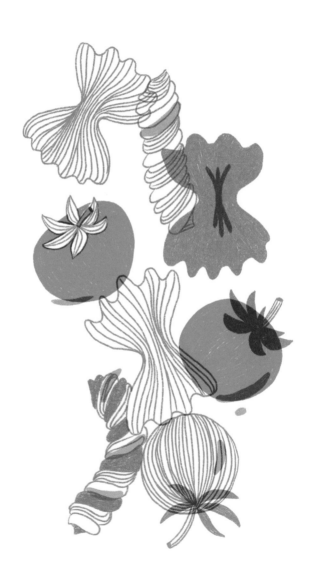

Feel Your Fullness

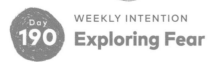

WEEKLY INTENTION
Exploring Fear

Diet culture pathologizes the feeling of fullness. Consequently, many people are afraid of this very natural cue that lets us know that we have had enough nourishment. Fullness is like the period at the end of a sentence—it's a natural stopping point.

This week: Explore if you are eating in a fearful and guarded way, like you're driving your car with one foot on the brake pedal. Do you cautiously stop eating before your true fullness point? (By the way, this is not necessarily a problem if you are willing to eat a little sooner to meet your body's needs.)

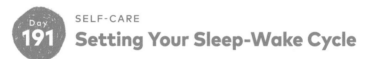

Day 191

SELF-CARE
Setting Your Sleep-Wake Cycle

Watching the sunrise and the sunset is a powerful way to set your sleep-wake cycle. (Important note—don't ever look directly at the sun because it can permanently damage your retinas.) It is as simple as viewing the

- Morning sunrise for two to ten minutes, ideally before 8:00 a.m.;
- Evening sunset for two to ten minutes, after 4:00 p.m.

Not only is this a beautiful way to start and end your day, it affects your circadian cycle by impacting the release of the hormones cortisol and melatonin. Promising research shows that doing this for only two days in a row is enough to reset your sleep-wake cycle.[19]

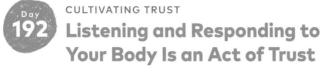

Day 192
Listening and Responding to Your Body Is an Act of Trust

Each time you judge yourself by an external standard, such as a scale, a food-tracking app, a mirror, or the opinion of others, you lose a little self-connection. Outsourcing your wants and needs moves you further away from your authentic self.

What's called for, instead, is a gentle yet radical shift to turning inward. This is a simple act of listening to your body, which is the gateway to getting to know your body and truly coming home. It's getting to know your needs from the inside.

Take a moment to check in with yourself, right now, to ask the universal attunement question. Overall, how do you feel right now? Pleasant, unpleasant, or neutral? Every time you check in with that simple question, you are listening and building trust.

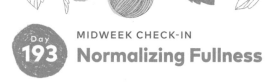

Normalizing Fullness

How are you doing with recognizing fullness? Is fear impacting when you choose to stop eating, perhaps masked by a sense of confusion? Getting to know fullness is an easier process when you are engaged in meal-based eating, rather than a grazing style of eating. There is no problem with either way of eating. But in the beginning, if you want more clarity in identifying fullness, it may be helpful to engage in more meal-based eating—substantial meals, typically three in a day with some snacks—rather than grazing on small frequent meals. That's because eating small frequent meals results in more nuanced levels of satiety cues, which can feel somewhat ambiguous.

Day
194

INTUITIVE EATING MANTRAS

Intuitive Eating is a pathway to body and food liberation.

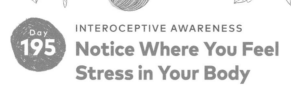

INTEROCEPTIVE AWARENESS

Day 195

Notice Where You Feel Stress in Your Body

It's so easy to lose touch with ourselves and our bodies during everyday life and its multitude of stresses—from catching up on never-ending emails to juggling a hectic schedule. We stay disconnected from our bodies, unless we check in.

PRACTICE
Today, during one of these frenetic times, take a moment to notice where you feel stress in your body. Perhaps it takes the form of a tight neck or a dull tension in your jaw or temples. Maybe it's a pit in your stomach. Or perhaps it's a sensation of tautness in your diaphragm that results in shallow breathing. Just notice. Every time you check in with your body, you learn more about yourself and build a bridge to self-connection.

BODY APPRECIATION

Day 196
Curate Radical Body Diversity on Social Media

We are born in diverse bodies. We were not all meant to have the same size, look, gender, or ability. Most mainstream media does not reflect, let alone celebrate, this incredible diversity. While there are many downsides to social media, there is a tremendous positive aspect. You can curate your feed to make it diverse—and more reflective of reality. Also, unfollowing can be just as powerful as following new accounts.

It helps to surround yourself with positive images of people leading fulfilling lives in diverse body shapes, sizes, genders, races, ages, and abilities. Check out and follow these accounts on Instagram:

@sonyareneetaylor
@fierce.fatty
@virgietovar
@antidietriotclub

@unlikelyhikers
@meg.boggs
@fatgirlstraveling
@mia.mingus

@jabbieapp
@brandonkgood
@iharterika
@drjcofthedc

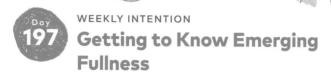

WEEKLY INTENTION
Getting to Know Emerging Fullness

You have been exploring fullness as a normal body sensation, which lets you know that you have nourished your body adequately. It's time to befriend this cue and tune in to the physical sensations of emerging fullness in your body. It's easy to miss emerging fullness, because in the beginning it's subtle, like a whisper.

One pleasant practice is to sip hot tea because it gives you a helpful focal point. Please note that the following exercise is not to trick your body to fake out hunger or to feel falsely full. Rather it's a practice to help guide your awareness toward the sensation of emerging fullness.

PRACTICE
Prepare enough hot water to make two to three cups of tea. Steep the tea to your liking. Begin sipping the tea, placing your awareness on the sensation of hot liquid traveling down your esophagus to your stomach. Notice how this feels. Continue drinking the tea until you actually feel the sensation of fullness in your stomach. (This may take two or three cups.) This fullness is temporary and fleeting. The sensation won't last very long because there is no sustenance in the tea.

This week: Using what you learned from the hot tea practice, place your awareness on emerging fullness during one of your meals.

Day 198

EMBODIED AFFIRMATIONS
I Am Able to Lean In to Difficult Feelings

It's important not to disregard your emotions. It's fine to temporarily distract yourself from them, but eventually, you'll need to experience your feelings. It can be particularly powerful to lean in to the bodily sensations of emotion, without engaging in the mental narrative or self-talk that usually accompanies them. While it might not feel this way, emotions are temporary. The more you try to repress an emotion, the longer it will be with you and likely overwhelm you. Allow yourself to be human and lean in to difficult emotions.

PRACTICE

Reflect on a time when you experienced a strong emotion, which eventually passed. (Please note, if this reflection feels too triggering, feel free to choose a different one.) Maybe it was when you cried at a funeral or felt intense disappointment from a rejection letter. When the situation is clear in your mind, place your awareness on the feeling of knowing you can handle difficult emotions.

Place your hand on your heart or in a self-hug, and slowly repeat three times, *"I am able to lean in to difficult feelings."*

Day 199

SELF-COMPASSION

Self-Compassion Is Not Toxic Positivity

While there are benefits to having positive thoughts or a bright outlook, it can problematic when this perspective glosses over or denies your reality. This is known as toxic positivity. At best, toxic positivity minimizes what you are going through, and at worst, it denies you the opportunity to build resilience. That's because it's a form of emotionally bypassing what you are really experiencing, which does not cultivate authentic self-connection.[20]

Self-compassion, on the other hand, is about connecting to and being with your suffering, while finding a warm, kind perspective. It's about having an inner best friend who offers a supportive kind voice, unconditionally.

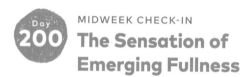

Day 200

MIDWEEK CHECK-IN

The Sensation of Emerging Fullness

It takes practice and focus to identify and feel emerging fullness. If this is difficult for you, that's okay. What's important is to cultivate patience and curiosity! It really is a practice to pay attention. Some people find it easier to continue using the hot tea practice (page 198) to help familiarize and focus their awareness on the felt sense of the body as it gets full.

Day
201

MEAL MEDITATIONS

Appreciating the Unfolding of My Progress

May I have compassion for eating-angst not yet healed.
May I have patience on my path toward Intuitive Eating.
May I blossom and have serenity at my plate.
May I recognize and appreciate my progress.

Day
202

INTUITIVE EATING MANTRAS

Sometimes, eating is ordinary, and that's okay.

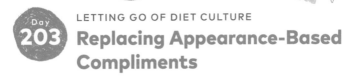

LETTING GO OF DIET CULTURE

Replacing Appearance-Based Compliments

Here are some nonappearance-based compliments that are more connected to a person's humanity:

- I love your energy.

- I admire how you live in alignment with your values.

- You seem really happy today.

- You are an amazing _____
  (friend, colleague, coworker, teacher, partner, teammate, ally, etc.).

- I admire your authenticity.

- I feel so comfortable around you.

- I feel really heard and safe with you.

- I appreciate your open-mindedness and ability to see multiple perspectives.

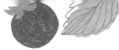
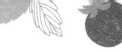
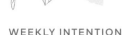

WEEKLY INTENTION

When You Are Pushed for Time: The Three-Bite Check-In

This Intuitive Eating check-in technique is handy when life is complicated, hurried, and stressful. While it would be optimal to eat your meals without distraction, it's not always possible. Rather than blowing off self-connection altogether, this practice asks you to give your undivided awareness to just three focused bites of food during a meal or snack. Please keep in mind that the following is just a practice, not another food rule!

This week: Choose one daily meal or snack to practice the three-bite check-in:

- *First bite:* Just before you take your first bite of food, check in with your body: How does your hunger feel overall—pleasant, unpleasant, or neutral? How does the food look, smell, and taste?

- *Middle bite:* In the middle of your meal, pause for the second intentional bite of food and notice: How does it taste? Is your hunger diminishing? Is there any emerging fullness?

- *Last bite:* When you finish eating your last bite of food, connect with your fullness level—is it pleasant, unpleasant, or neutral?

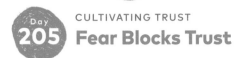

CULTIVATING TRUST

Fear Blocks Trust

Fear blocks your inborn ability to trust your body's wisdom. Sadly, we live in a fearmongering world, which instills a sense that you are one bite away from disaster. Our culture has given too much power to food, and, in doing so, has robbed us of the joy of eating. Unless you have a lethal food allergy, eating a particular food will not kill you. Remember that one food, meal, or day will not make or break your health.

LOVING BOUNDARIES

Yes, You Can Love Your Family AND Still Need to Set Boundaries

Diet culture primes a lot of people to think in binary terms—pass or fail, good or bad, on or off a diet. Setting boundaries is not black and white. You can still love someone AND need to set a boundary around diet talk or body comments. They are not mutually exclusive.

- I love my mom, and I need to set a boundary around her body comments.

- I love my dad, and I need set a boundary around his food comments directed at me.

- I love my sister, and I need to set a boundary around her diet talk.

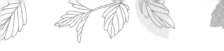
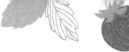
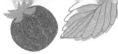

Day 207

MIDWEEK CHECK-IN

What Have You Noticed about Your Fullness?

What patterns have you noticed about your fullness? If you stopped at pleasant fullness, what factors helped you recognize it? If you ended up experiencing unpleasant fullness, what might you do differently next time? Check in with your body a little sooner? Remember, eating past fullness is not a failure—it's a learning opportunity that helps you get to know your body better! Eating past fullness from time to time is also part of normal eating.

Day 208

SELF-CARE

Permission to Play

When was the last time you played, spontaneously, just for the heck of it? Play is so important to our well-being—but when life gets complicated, our play tends to fizzle out.

Give yourself permission to play! Try something that sounds fun to you, perhaps one of these: blow bubbles, swing at a park or school, walk in water, splash in puddles, make art with sidewalk chalk, ride a bike, play a board game, play cards, dance, or build a sandcastle. The options really are endless!

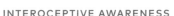

INTEROCEPTIVE AWARENESS

The Gift of Unpleasant Body Sensations

What if you viewed unpleasant body sensations as a gift for getting your basic needs met? An inconvenient gift, perhaps. Sometimes, you might not like the physical message from your body, such as

- A pounding heart rate and a physical restlessness, which perhaps reflect fear and a need for soothing;

- Heavy eyelids and weary, heavy limbs, which may reflect the need to take a rest, a break, or even a nap;

- A throbbing dull pain in your tooth, which might signal the need to see the appropriate health-care professional.

Sometimes, if you disregard a message, the body sensations get louder—like someone pounding on your door trying to get your attention, saying, "Please let me in!" What might you need to let in today?

Day
210

INTUITIVE EATING MANTRAS

Intuitive Eating is my path
to freedom, away from
diet culture.

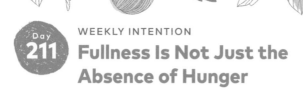

WEEKLY INTENTION

Fullness Is Not Just the Absence of Hunger

As you get to know your body and the sensations of fullness, there is a nuance that's important to discern. When you are hungry and begin eating a meal, you will get to a point where hunger is no longer present. But this is NOT fullness. Rather, it's the absence of hunger.

For example, suppose you are super hungry, and you sit down to a bowl of chili and cornbread. Halfway through the chili, you might notice that your hunger pangs are gone. Yet if you were to stop eating at that point, you would likely feel a sense of incompleteness and a desire to continue eating. That's appropriate! That's why if you decided to stop eating at the point of absence of hunger, rather than fullness, you will feel hungry sooner.

This week: When you are eating meals, pause at the midpoint (this does not need to be exact). Notice the sensations you are feeling, hunger-wise. It is common to feel ambiguity, where there is neither a clear hunger nor clear fullness. (That's a sensation too!) Make a mental note of this experience. When you finish eating, note your fullness level. How do you feel now compared to how you felt at the midpoint? Notice the difference. Keep in mind that this is a direct experience, not an intellectual exercise. The feelings of hunger and fullness are dynamic and may manifest in various ways. This is an ongoing practice, not a box to check off and leave behind.

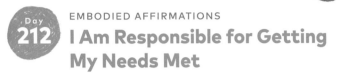

EMBODIED AFFIRMATIONS

Day 212

I Am Responsible for Getting My Needs Met

Only you can be the expert on you and your needs. Nobody could possibly know what you feel. You might need to end a night out with friends earlier than intended because you're tired. Or you might need to decline a project because you already have too many responsibilities.

PRACTICE

Recall a time when you declined to take on an important responsibility or project. Perhaps you didn't have the bandwidth to do a good job or simply didn't have it in you because you had too many other competing obligations. Did you feel relief after you declined? Now intensify this feeling of relief, or knowingness, about not being able to take on one more thing.

Using this feeling, with your hand on your heart or in a self-hug, slowly repeat three times, *"I am responsible for getting my needs met."*

BODY APPRECIATION
Aliveness of My Heart

Place your hand on your vibrant heart. Can you feel your heart beating? Consider that this beautiful organ throbs over and over, just for you. Through thick and thin, your heart keeps ticking. Over the course of one year, the average human heart will pulsate from about thirty-one to more than fifty-three billion beats![21]

Can you shift your perspective to the inside of your body for appreciation and gratitude, for your one-and-only beating heart?

MIDWEEK CHECK-IN
Distinguishing Absence of Hunger from Fullness

Have you been able to identify and feel the difference between the absence of hunger and comfortable fullness? This nuanced awareness of these sensations would be hard to access if you eat while multitasking (like watching TV or reading). It might be a while before you can distinguish these sensations, and that's okay. Please be patient and kind with yourself.

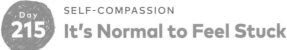

SELF-COMPASSION

Day 215

It's Normal to Feel Stuck

Even when you are clear that you want to leave diet culture for good, you can still feel quite stuck. On one hand, you may feel terrified to move forward on the path of Intuitive Eating. And on the other hand, you are very clear that you cannot continue living the way you have been, steeped in diet culture, worried about every morsel of food you put into your mouth, constantly preoccupied with what you are going to eat next, and checked out of life. This is a very common place to find yourself, and it does not feel good. Please know that this is expected. Of course, you are scared— change is scary. This is completely normal.

PRACTICE
How can you kindly support yourself if and when you are feeling stuck?

LETTING GO OF DIET CULTURE

Acknowledging Short-Term Relief, at the Expense of Long-Term Suffering

It's really common to get lured into the just-one-more-try-to-shrink-my-body trap. It's often a lingering fantasy flickering in the back of your mind, which means the diet mentality is still present. (It's so understandable with diet culture surrounding you everywhere you go). This is where it's helpful to reflect on what your lived experience has shown you. Sure, you might have lost weight in the short run. But what about over time? Research confirms that dieting is not sustainable and negatively impacts the quality of your life.[22]

It's helpful to acknowledge that diet culture behaviors, by whatever name you call them, are a short-term relief, which usher in long-time suffering. Where have you seen this in your own life?

Day 217

CULTIVATING TRUST
Consistent Acts of Self-Kindness Repair Trust

If you had a friend who often flaked out on you, would you trust that friend? Probably not! In order for a relationship to flourish, there needs to be a safe bond where both parties can rely on each other. Relationships are mutually interdependent, including the one you have with your body.

Can your body rely on you to treat it well? When you loathe your body or feel that your body is not good enough, it's really common to treat it unkindly. If your body relationship is fraught with running it into the ground, withholding food, or ignoring the messages that it sends you, then it's hard to expect a consistent response from your body (such as hunger, fullness, and satisfaction). Body chaos disrupts self-connection and trust.

Each time you meet a need of your body, like nourishment, rest, or attuned movement, you are repairing trust, one act of self-kindness at a time. It's consistency, not perfection, that matters.

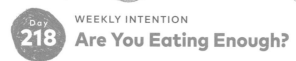

WEEKLY INTENTION

Are You Eating Enough?

If you tend to eat a lot of vegetables at a meal, like in an entrée salad, you might notice a conflicting feeling of simultaneous fullness and incompleteness. That's because the volume and fiber from the veggies trigger the fullness receptors in the stomach, but that's only part of where fullness gets registered in your body. It's also managed by your brain and nervous system.

Your body is very smart, which is why you may still want more food, even though you feel full. This can also happen while dieting: You fill up on foods that have a lot of volume, but lack sufficient energy or calories. Consequently, you think about food a lot sooner and more frequently.

If you find you are hungry two or three hours after a meal, that could be a sign that you are not eating enough food during that meal. (This is not a problem as long as you don't mind honoring your hunger more frequently throughout the day.) In general, if you have eaten enough food at a meal, it will sustain you for about four to six hours.

This can also happen with snacks. You may eat an apple, for example, and then experience hunger thirty minutes to an hour later. This could be an indication that the snack wasn't enough to sustain you until your next meal.

This week: Notice if you have experiences with incomplete fullness, feeling somewhat full and still wanting to eat—whether you want a full meal or a snack.

Day
219

INTUITIVE EATING MANTRAS

The journey of Intuitive Eating takes time, patience, and self-kindness.

Day 220

Recognizing Reactivity

We can't control our initial emotions or root thoughts, but we can manage our reactions to them. Reactivity is an automatic response to a situation, thought, or feeling. It can happen so fast, it's easy to miss. Reactivity is not intentional or thoughtful: rather it's a knee-jerk reaction.

When it comes to eating and body-related issues, reactive behavior can look like this:

- Deciding you ate too much at a meal and skipping meals for the rest of the day.

- Eating dessert and automatically compensating by "working it off" with more exercise.

- Vowing to eat less when you feel that your body is unacceptable.

- Perceiving that you ate the "wrong" food or the "wrong" amount and compensating by eating less the next day.

This pattern becomes one of compensatory actions—like starting a new food plan or program, or working out more, without regard to what your body needs and feels.

Sometimes, if the process of Intuitive Eating doesn't feel like it's progressing fast enough, there's a tendency to want to jump into just one more food plan. This is where the work is—practicing not reacting to disappointment. Recognizing this compensatory reflex pattern is the way forward, an opportunity to work through uncomfortable feelings about your eating and your body differently.

MIDWEEK CHECK-IN
Nuances of Fullness

What have you noticed so far around the nuances of fullness? The more you understand the intricacies of how food feels in your body, the more you will be able to dial in and match your body's daily needs in everyday life.

Day
222

SELF-CARE
Pause

An important part of self-care is the ability to tune in with how you feel, because it helps you figure out what you need. It's like when you get in the driver's seat of the car and check the instrument panel; what's the status of your car? For example, is there enough gas to get to your destination?

PRACTICE
Pause and check in with yourself. How do you feel in this moment? Pleasant, unpleasant, or neutral? Based on the answer to this question, what might you need to do today to honor your self-care?

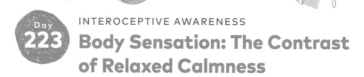

Day 223

INTEROCEPTIVE AWARENESS

Body Sensation: The Contrast of Relaxed Calmness

The following is a series of practices that will have you tighten or clench parts of your body for a few seconds, alternating with relaxing that body part for the same amount of time. Take a relaxed seated position and engage in the following:

1. Scrunch up your face and hold the tension for a few seconds, then relax it.

2. Tighten your fists, then relax them.

3. Tighten your chest and arms, then relax them.

4. Clench your abdomen, then relax it.

5. Clench your butt, then relax it.

6. Tighten your legs, then relax them.

7. Bunch up and clench your feet, then relax them.

Now, tighten your entire body from head to toe. Hold it for about five seconds. Next, completely relax your entire body from head to toe. From the inside out, place your awareness on the whole felt sense of your body. How would you describe it? (See the list of descriptions on p. 65.)

Day 224

MEAL MEDITATIONS

Where Does Your Mind Go When You Eat?

As I nourish my body with the food set before me,
I will gently cultivate awareness of my thoughts.
How often am I lost in thought?
When I become aware that I'm lost in thought,
I'll kindly redirect my mind to one of my favorite sensations of eating—
Taste, sight, smell, touch, swallowing, or aftertaste.

Cope with Your Emotions with Kindness

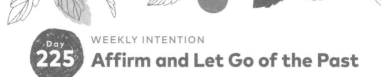

Day 225

Affirm and Let Go of the Past

We all eat for comfort from time to time—that's part of normal eating. For many people, turning to food for solace in seasons of crisis or trauma is the only option for emotional survival. There is no shame in that. It's important to recognize and pay homage to yourself with kindness for finding a way to cope the best way that you could, with the resources that you had at the time.

Also, keep in mind that when you add dieting or any kind of food restriction to the mix, there seems to be an added biological drive to eat during emotional duress.[23]

This week: While it's important to have a variety of coping tools, the practice this week is to affirm the role that food has had in your emotional life and let go of any judgment or, especially, shame. What would you say to a dear friend or loved one who has used food to self-soothe and cope with emotions?

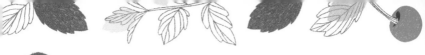

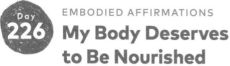

EMBODIED AFFIRMATIONS

My Body Deserves to Be Nourished

Thanks to diet culture, it's easy to get the idea that you are eating "too much" or that you don't deserve to eat according to your own hunger and satisfied fullness. This might mean you eat more than other people at a meal or an event. There's nothing wrong with that—only you know what your body needs!

PRACTICE

Recall a time in which you were really hungry and ate enough food to feel nourished and satisfied. Remember the contented feeling and how it affected your energy, ability to focus, and mood. Now intensify this feeling of being nourished adequately and feeling energized.

Using this feeling, with your hand on your heart or in a self-hug, slowly repeat three times, *"My body deserves to be nourished."*

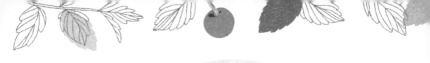

Day
227

INTUITIVE EATING MANTRAS

Trusting the process of Intuitive Eating takes time.

Day
228

MIDWEEK CHECK-IN
Letting Go of Judgment and Shame

Letting go of judgment and shame is an important step toward healing. This acknowledges that you do the best that you can, with the tools available to you at the time. The more complex your history, such as past trauma, eating disorder, dieting, food insecurity, or any combination thereof, the longer it may take to cultivate new and varied tools to cope with difficult emotions. That's okay—this is part of the healing.

CULTIVATING TRUST
Your Lived Experience

"Experience is, for me, the highest authority. The touchstone of validity is my own experience. No other person's ideas and none of my own ideas are as authoritative as my experience. It is to experience that I must return again and again, to discover a closer approximation to truth . . ."

—CARL ROGERS, *ON BECOMING A PERSON* [24]

Your lived experiences are an invaluable part of cultivating a healthy relationship with food, mind, and body. These are more powerful than any study or statistic that I, or anyone else, could offer you. Noticing and reflecting on the experiences of your body is part of your pathway to healing. There is ultimate freedom when validation and knowledge come from within. Consider

- *Your body's experience of losing control from being too hungry on a food plan.* That's your experience of your body working and protecting you from what it perceives as starvation. That's dieting failing you.

- *Feeling cranky and irritable from not getting enough to eat while on a diet.* That's your mind's experience of and response to undereating.

- *Your mind's fixation on food when you are on a restrictive food plan.* That's your mind's attempt to stay alive; it's a mental food-seeking survival mechanism.

- *Your mind's preoccupation with the size of your body.* That's one of the harmful effects of the constant, culturally sanctioned fat phobia that surrounds us.

You are not broken; our weight-obsessed culture is part of your learned conditioning. When you start to notice how your body and mind feel with consistent and unconditional nourishment, it becomes a powerful lived experience. Your truth.

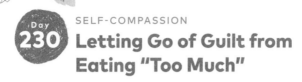

Day 230 Letting Go of Guilt from Eating "Too Much"

Eating too much means different things to different people. Through the lens of kindness, explore these questions to help you process and let go of the guilt:

- *Is it possible that your body needed this food?* Sometimes we have hungrier days.

- *Did you have an unmet need that wasn't addressed? Perhaps you needed a break or basic self-care?*

- *Is it possible that you went too long since eating your last meal?* In these situations, you become urgently hungry, and with this primal hunger, it's really easy to bypass comfortable fullness.

- *Were you connected to your body and the experience of eating, or were you disconnected and checked out?* Perhaps you deemed overeating as "wrong" or "bad" and to bypass the feeling of guilt or shame you disengaged with the experience of eating.

- *What can you learn from this experience?* Learning from your experience helps you let go.

- *Last, what would you say to a dear friend who was struggling with a similar situation?*

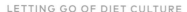

Diet culture and all its related products and services is the only industry that blames the consumer for poor or temporary outcomes! The sad part is that consumers believe they are indeed at fault—that they didn't try hard enough or long enough. This mind-bending victim blaming is known as *gaslighting*, which is aptly named after the movie *Gaslight*. This classic thriller, starring Ingrid Bergman, is about a husband who manipulates and tricks his wife into thinking she is losing her mind. Diet culture does the same. You are not lacking willpower, discipline, or strength. Diet culture is the problem, not you.

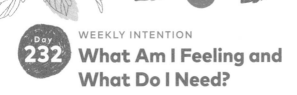

WEEKLY INTENTION
What Am I Feeling and What Do I Need?

An important part of self-connection is getting to know how your emotions feel both physically and psychologically. If you have been in the habit of avoiding or denying your feelings, this will take ongoing practice of checking in.

This week: Get curious, without judgment, and notice where in your body you experience different emotions. (In the beginning, it is easier to recognize intense emotions.) What is the quality of the emotion—pleasant, unpleasant, or neutral?

If you find yourself turning to food during uncomfortable feelings, try asking yourself: What am I feeling right now—and what might I need right now related to this feeling? Don't expect an answer right away; it's a process that takes curiosity and patience.

Day 233

Letting Go of the Exasperating Project of Changing Your Body

"There is more reason in your body than in your best wisdom."

—NIETZSCHE[25]

Contrary to deeply rooted beliefs propagated by diet culture, body size is not a choice! Your weight is regulated by a complex set of powerful factors *beyond your conscious control*, which include genetics, biology, gut microbiome, social determinants, and more.

There is a profound body of scientific evidence showing that the pursuit of weight loss through dieting is not sustainable for the vast majority of people—upward of 95 percent of diets fail! Furthermore, food restriction harms health by increasing the risk of eating disorders, weight stigma, weight cycling, depression, body dissatisfaction, and anxiety.[26]

Day 234

Feeling Guilty for Setting Boundaries

If you are not used to letting people know what's okay and not okay with you, setting boundaries can feel unsettling at first. Sometimes you might feel twinges of guilt if you tend to be a people pleaser. But when you try to keep everyone in your life happy at the expense of your needs, it really is not healthy for you! Keep in mind that when you are choosing to set boundaries, you are choosing

- Authentic communication over silence, which prevents growing resentment;

- To protect your vital limited energy, which prevents burnout and compassion fatigue;

- Self-respect, which teaches others how to treat you;

- To model healthy communication.

Day 235

Getting Your Needs Met

Simply asking the question, "What do I need right now?" is therapeutic in and of itself. It's a gentle acknowledgment and reminder that you have needs. If you are used to putting other people's needs ahead of yours, this question might feel daunting. There is nothing wrong with being of service to other people and causes. The problem is when you do so at the expense of taking care of yourself.

Day 236

INTUITIVE EATING MANTRAS

The shape and size of my body is not a reflection of my worthiness.

Silencing Ruminating Thoughts

Listening to the sensations of your body helps you meet your emotional and physical needs—but there is also a very important secondary benefit. It silences ruminating thoughts, which is a closed-loop pattern of anxiety-provoking thinking and endless mind-stories that tend to be negative.[27] This type of thinking does not get you anywhere except to incessant worry.

Placing your awareness on body sensations gives your mind a focal point: the here-and-now moment, which simultaneously dampens ruminating thoughts.

PRACTICE
The next time you find yourself absorbed in a story line or ruminating thoughts, place your attention on the sensation of your beating heart or the sensation of your body breathing (choose whichever feels the most accessible in the moment). Notice the incessant thoughts subside as your concentration intensifies.

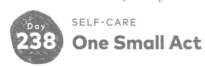

Day 238
One Small Act

What's one small act of self-care or self-kindness that you could engage in today? Self-care is an important part of our health, but most of us have not been taught to value it. It really is a practice. What sounds appealing to you?

- Take a short nap.

- Take a walk around the block.

- Give yourself a small transition break, say five minutes, after arriving home from school, work, or a meeting. Sit in the car, or at the bus stop or train station, before going inside. Perhaps just close your eyes and do nothing.

- Turn off your phone for thirty minutes.

- Stretch or do yoga for five minutes.

- Watch the sunset.

- Journal or doodle for five minutes.

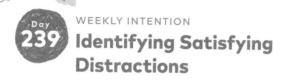

WEEKLY INTENTION

Identifying Satisfying Distractions

Sometimes you need a break from your emotions, especially the chronic ones that seem unrelenting, like worrying if you will get hired or have to move for a new job. It's important to not only identify your emotions so that you know what you are feeling to get your needs met, but to also find satisfying distractions when you need a time-out from your feelings. (Note that this is different from chronic avoidance of feelings, which could be problematic.)

This week: Consider what could be sources of engaging distractions for you—things that have the qualities of absorbing your attention without causing you to feel worse after engaging in them. For example, compulsive shopping might be alluring and exciting but could put your finances in harm's way, which will leave you feeling lousy in the long run. A positive, satisfying distraction might be curating puppy videos on Instagram or YouTube, planning a vacation, reading an absorbing book, or engaging in a creative project.

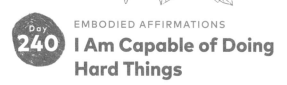

EMBODIED AFFIRMATIONS

Day 240 I Am Capable of Doing Hard Things

Diet and food plan cycling can erode self-confidence. This affirmation will help remind you of your capabilities.

PRACTICE

Recall a time when you were faced with a challenging situation and overcame it. Perhaps it was when you were a child, maybe a teen. Perhaps it was a recent event. Maybe it was finishing something, like school, a project, therapy, or recovery of some sort. It doesn't have to be a big event; what's important is that it felt significant and empowering for you. Connect with the feeling of getting through a tough situation; perhaps there was a sense of pride or determinedness. Now amplify that feeling.

Using this feeling, and with your hand on your heart or in a self-hug, slowly repeat three times, "*I am capable of doing hard things.*"

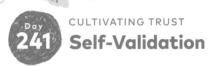

Day 241

CULTIVATING TRUST
Self-Validation

How often do you rely on others for validation? Seeking external approval from others obscures self-trust. Self-trust is like the sun residing inside you. Each time you look to others instead of yourself, it becomes clouded over. Over time, this perpetuates indecision, self-doubt, and fear of failure. Know that the ability to reawaken self-trust is within in you. It's similar to a stormy day; we know that the sun exists—even if hidden by blustery clouds.

What would it look like to seek wisdom, validation, and truth from within yourself? What am I feeling? What do I need today? What feels right for me at this moment?

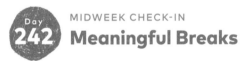

Day 242

MIDWEEK CHECK-IN
Meaningful Breaks

As you experiment with different ways to get a time-out from uncomfortable feelings, you will start to learn what works and what doesn't. This only comes from experience, which cultivates self-knowledge. It's like trying on shoes. Shoes can look great—but sometimes when you wear them and walk around, they just don't feel right. They're a nice style, perhaps, but not a match for what you need. That's okay.

Day 243
Self-Compassion's Ripple Effect

Self-compassion is not indulgent or selfish—it's quite the opposite. A delightful benefit of self-compassion is that as you cultivate more compassion for yourself, you develop more compassion for other people in the process!

Day 244

INTUITIVE EATING MANTRAS

I am honoring the inner GPS of my body signals.

Day 245

Creating a Safe Space for Body Sacredness at Home

Wouldn't it be wonderful if your home was truly your sanctuary—for you and all bodies who enter it—a safe zone, free from body denigration? This begins with acknowledging that all bodies are worthy of respect and dignity. With that in mind, you could let people know that "My home is a diet culture–free space, in which all bodies are sacred. Therefore all who enter are asked to abide by the following":

- Do not comment on anyone's body, including your own. (This includes compliments and criticisms.)

- Do not weigh or measure your body (unless there is medical necessity).

- If guests initiate body-talk, you will kindly ask them to honor your body sanctuary boundaries.

We cannot change culture overnight, but we can create a safe respite in our homes for all bodies who enter.

Day 246

WEEKLY INTENTION
Who Are Your Connections?

Who are your go-to people when you need emotional support, or just a sounding board to hold space when you are feeling distressed? You might have lots of friends on social media, but who are the people you can trust with difficult emotions?

This week: Take inventory of your personal relationships. Do you have people in your inner circle who you can open up to, whom you trust with your deep emotions? If the answer is no, what could you do to start cultivating these types of intimate relationships, knowing that they don't happen overnight?

Day 247

MEAL MEDITATIONS
Sacred Traditions

May I honor the sacred bonding of life's
celebrations and milestones through food.
May I appreciate the eating traditions and
cuisines of my culture and my ancestors.
May I respect the connections that food brings.
May I enjoy the pleasures of the palate.

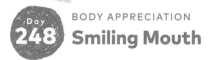

BODY APPRECIATION
Day 248
Smiling Mouth

Thank you to my mouth—for allowing me to smile and connect with loved ones, friends, and strangers. My smile lets me share joy with a well-timed joke or witty remark. My smile offers a wordless reassurance: It's going to be okay. My smile communicates a sense of glowing satisfaction for a job well-done. My smile offers an affirming welcome—it's so good to see you; or come here, and sit by me.

What do you appreciate about your smile?

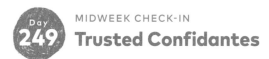

MIDWEEK CHECK-IN
Day 249
Trusted Confidantes

How are you doing with identifying trusted confidantes? Is it possible there are safe people in your life, but you don't feel comfortable opening up? If that's the case, what might you need in order to feel safe connecting with others in this way?

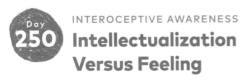

Day 250

Intellectualization Versus Feeling

It's easy to get caught up living in your head—like eating according to the rigid rules of a food plan, instead of attuning with your personal appetite and satisfaction. This can also happen with emotions. Rather than feeling emotions, both in the body and psychologically, there can be a tendency to intellectualize. Intellectualization blocks out the experience of *feeling* emotions by focusing on just the logic and facts of a situation. It's a common defense mechanism, which often starts with these phases:

- Using thought descriptions such as "I think . . ." as opposed to "I feel . . ."

- Using descriptors of how you think you should be feeling, which can bypass your actual emotions, such as "I should feel grateful . . . ," when you are actually feeling disappointed.

- Using metaphors, like "I'm spread too thin," that describe the situation but not how you feel, such as overwhelmed.

The work-around is to get curious and notice. What am I feeling in my body? What am I feeling emotionally?

Day 251

INTUITIVE EATING MANTRAS

Nourishment as self-care supports my Intuitive Eating if and when my satiety cues are offline because of stress, illness, or other circumstances.

Day 252

Getting Comfortable with Uncertainty

Paradoxically, uncertainty is one of the most certain aspects of life, because nobody knows exactly what's going to happen in the future. Humans don't handle this notion very well, even though most of us intellectually understand the truism of uncertainty. So when diet culture swoops in with promises of weight loss, it is dangling the seductive (but untrue) carrot of certainty.

Embracing uncertainty with a true knowingness that whatever happens, *I got this*, helps cultivate trust. How would it feel to say to yourself, *There isn't anything I can't handle; whatever happens, I got this*?

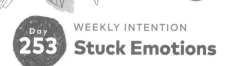

Day 253 **Stuck Emotions**

When experiencing an unpleasant emotion, it is not uncommon to have a distorted sense of time, one that seems frozen and everlasting. While we may intellectually know that no emotion is permanent, it can certainly feel that way in the moment!

According to Harvard-trained neuroanatomist Dr. Jill Bolte Taylor, the longest duration of an emotion physiologically is ninety seconds.[28] Does that sound preposterous? Keep in mind that the story you tell yourself about the emotion keeps the feeling alive in your body.

This week: When you are feeling an uncomfortable emotion, practice this technique. Identify your emotion. Just observe. Detect where you feel it in your body and *how long it lasts*. Here's the tricky part—notice without getting stuck in a story or narrative as to how or why you are feeling the emotion. The moment you become aware that you are getting lost in your thoughts or the story, shift your awareness back to your body, the place where you are experiencing the emotion. Notice when you experience a shift in the intensity of the feeling.

EMBODIED AFFIRMATIONS

My Body Is a Sacred Gift

We live in a culture that criticizes, shames, and denigrates our bodies—without any positive regard to the miracle of life they truly are. This affirmation will remind you of the sacredness of having a body.

PRACTICE

Recall a time when you were in awe of your body. Perhaps it was healing from an injury or illness, growing inches in a single year, or giving birth to a baby. Connect with the feeling of awe or sacredness. Now amplify that feeling.

Place your hand on your heart or in a self-hug and slowly repeat three times, *"My body is a sacred gift."*

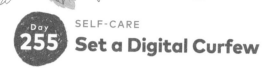

Day 255

Set a Digital Curfew

Most of us use electronic devices up until bedtime. The problem is that these devices are stimulating and disrupt the natural release of our sleep hormone, melatonin. This makes it harder to fall asleep and stay asleep.

The National Sleep Foundation recommends establishing a digital curfew—optimally, about two hours before bed.[29] The earlier the better, but initiating a realistic digital curfew is what really matters, even if you shut everything down only thirty minutes before you go to bed.

To get into the routine, try setting an alarm to remind you to turn off your electronics. Notice how this feels. Try winding down by reading a physical book or journaling on paper.

MIDWEEK CHECK-IN

Day 256

Temporary Nature of Emotions

Connecting with your body to help identify your emotions is a valuable practice. You can do this any time because no matter where you are, you have access to awareness. What was the longest period of time that you experienced an emotion? It's helpful and kind to remind ourselves that the emotion will pass, and so will its intensity.

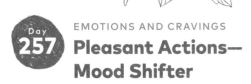

Day 257

Pleasant Actions—Mood Shifter

Sometimes, we need a quick pick-me-up to allow our mood to shift a little easier. I also want to be clear—this is not about bypassing our feelings. It's important to experience emotions for our mental health. But sometimes we need a little shift, and that's okay too. Try any one of these pleasant actions to see if they create a lightening of your spirits:

- Do one random act of kindness, such as opening a door for a stranger or buying someone a cup of coffee.

- Send a gratitude text to a friend or family member.

- Take three relaxing breaths.

- Play with a puppy or kitten.

- Watch an online comedy performance.

- Watch an uplifting or inspiring movie.

- Step outside for fresh air.

- Other _____.

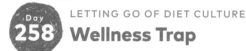

LETTING GO OF DIET CULTURE

Day 258

Wellness Trap

There's nothing wrong with wanting to support your health through your food choices. However, the wellness industry and its social media influencers peddle "wellness" as another form of diet culture, profiting off insecurities and promising everlasting health through supplements and rigid ways of eating. The problem is that the pursuit of so-called "healthy eating" often comes at the expense of your psychological and social well-being.

When a person becomes obsessed with healthy eating, it's called *orthorexia*. This rigid way of eating with lots of food rules is paradoxically unhealthy. While orthorexia is not yet recognized as an official medical diagnosis, many health professionals classify it as a form of eating disorder. Sadly, research indicates that a significant proportion of the healthy eating community on Instagram has orthorexic symptoms.[30]

Unless you have a life-threatening allergy to food, like peanuts, or a disease, such as celiac disease, food rules generally cause more harm than good. This also holds true for the wellness trap. The pursuit of rigid so-called healthy behaviors occupies an inordinate amount of time, energy, money, and headspace, ultimately distracting you from fully engaging in life outside the kitchen.

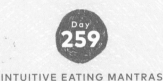

Day
259

INTUITIVE EATING MANTRAS

I am working on observing
my thoughts, feelings,
and body sensations
with nonjudgmental
awareness.

Respect Your Body

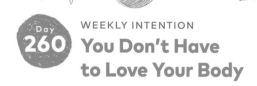

WEEKLY INTENTION
You Don't Have to Love Your Body

You don't have to love your body in order to respect it. Body respect comes from the inside out—it's not about your appearance. It's an attitude of unconditional positive regard for your humanity, period. Dignity and respect are your birthright as a sentient being.

You can still struggle with loving your body, and that's okay. Many people have spent a lifetime internalizing societal and family beliefs about what a body "should" look like. It's important to give yourself grace, and be patient with the process of healing your relationship with your body. In the meantime, you can still practice acts of body respect.

This week: From the following list, choose one activity to practice daily:

I will treat my body with respect by_____

- Speaking kindly to myself.
- Giving myself permission to take a nap or a break.
- Allowing myself to leave a toxic conversation about dieting or how bodies should look.
- Getting adequate sleep (seven to nine hours per night).
- Wearing comfortable shoes.
- Taking a relaxing bath.
- Not postponing my life until my body changes the way it looks.
- Going out with friends.

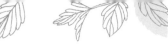

 Day 261

SELF-COMPASSION
Falling into Seductive Diet Traps

It's common to get ensnared in a diet trap, even when you are trying to cultivate a healthy relationship with food, mind, and body. Rather than get angry with yourself for not being a "perfect" Intuitive Eater (spoiler alert—that doesn't exist!), it's a great opportunity to practice self-compassion during these times. Consider:

- You are not alone with these experiences—diet culture is fierce and insidious.

- There is no such thing as a perfect Intuitive Eater.

- Perhaps this little misstep gave you the lived experience you needed to really know, once and for all, that dieting doesn't work—no matter how shiny diet culture or its influencers package it.

- What valuable lesson did you learn from this experience?

Approaching an experience through the lens of self-compassion and learning helps you let go. This perspective allows your mistakes to transcend into wisdom.

Day 262

Grounding: Like a Deeply Rooted Giant Redwood Tree

Grounding yourself helps you stay self-connected in the present, which is a necessary part of interoceptive awareness and Intuitive Eating. When a big gusty storm blows through a forest of giant redwood trees, their leaves and branches may shake—but the roots remain firmly and deeply embedded. So whether your storm condition consists of being overwhelmed by emotions, an unexpected event, or receiving disappointing news, know that it's temporary. This too shall pass. With deeply planted roots, you will survive the feeling of being overwhelmed by your emotions. Remember, emotions are not good or bad, but valuable opportunities to tune in to your body and get your needs met.

MIDWEEK CHECK-IN

Day 263

Acts of Body Respect

How are your acts of body respect coming along? You are in charge of how you speak to yourself and how you take care of yourself. Have you discovered more ways to treat your body respectfully?

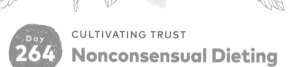

CULTIVATING TRUST
Nonconsensual Dieting

"Nonconsensual dieting" is a brilliant term coined by clinical social worker Sonalee Rashatwar, LCSW MEd. Essentially, this is when parents put a child on a food-restriction plan for the purpose of weight loss. Children have neither the capacity nor understanding to consent to food restrictions and rules. (Note, this is not about shaming well-meaning parents; it's about the impact and problems that ensue.)

There are long-term implications of nonconsensual dieting during childhood because it's a profound disruptor of basic autonomy. It sends the harmful message to the child that they cannot be trusted around food—that there is inherently something wrong with their body.

When kids are denied access to adequate food, the very natural feeling of hunger can become scary and confusing. They may eat to uncomfortable fullness when food is available, or they may lose the ability to discern what hunger and fullness feel like in their bodies altogether. It's not uncommon for kids in this situation to hide or sneak food, especially the kinds of food that their parents or guardians prohibit them from eating.

If this was your upbringing, please know that healing is possible, but it will likely take longer because the seeds of self-doubt were planted at such an early age.

BODY APPRECIATION

Making Peace with Your Body: Healing Doesn't Happen in the Mirror

If you have been conditioned to measure your self-worth by the way you look and by the size of your body, you will be perpetually unhappy because appearance and bodies change. Your inherent value comes from within—that's why healing doesn't happen in the mirror. It's about shifting your perspective and rejecting the image-obsessed cultural conditioning. Healing happens in the mind.

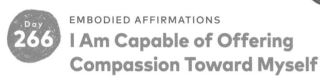

Day 266

I Am Capable of Offering Compassion Toward Myself

The internalized unforgiving and judgmental mindset of diet culture can be uprooted through the practice of self-compassion, which is pivotal for healing your relationship with food, mind, and body. If you are capable of extending compassion to others, you are capable of extending it to yourself. It's just a matter of shifting the direction inward.

PRACTICE

Recall a time when you offered compassion to another person. Perhaps it was toward your child, a friend, a dear relative, or a coworker. If you can, remember the words you offered. When this situation is recollected in your mind, connect with the feeling of compassionately knowing what to do. Amplify this feeling.

Then place your hand on your heart or in a self-hug and slowly repeat three times, *"I am capable of offering compassion toward myself."*

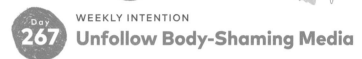

Day 267

Unfollow Body-Shaming Media

It's time to let go of media that disrespects bodies—any body type. Bodies come in diverse shapes, sizes, and weights. But that might not be so evident when perusing magazine covers or looking at the leading roles in movies and television shows.

This week: First, notice any media that triggers body shame, body comparison, or general insecurity about your body. This includes television, newspapers, magazines, podcasts, and books. (Hopefully you already curated your social media feed on Day 15.) Unsubscribe from people, organizations, or accounts that criticize or gossip about bodies, show before and after pictures, or show physique pictures. Other bodies are not a reflection of what you should or should not look like—your body is unique, and that's worthy of celebration!

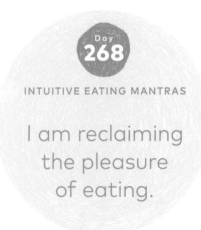

Day 268

INTUITIVE EATING MANTRAS

I am reclaiming
the pleasure
of eating.

Day 269

LOVING BOUNDARIES
Setting Boundaries for Yourself

Setting boundaries for yourself is a form of self-care and self-respect. Which of these boundaries resonate with you? For the most part, I

- Honor my hunger, even when others around me don't feel like eating.
- Take time to feel and process my emotions, rather than minimize or bypass them.
- Honor my needs, without explanation or apology.
- Take time for myself, whether it's via a break, a nap, or a day off from socializing.
- Make spiritual practices a priority.
- Limit my time with people who drain me.
- Don't participate in toxic conversations, which can include diet culture or gossip.
- Make time to eat without distraction, when possible and desired.
- Honor my financial commitments, which can include starting or maintaining an emergency savings fund or turning down an invitation to eat out with friends.

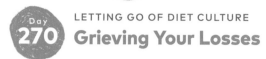

Grieving Your Losses

To make room for living life at the fullest, free from the toxicity of diet culture, it's healing and healthy to grieve for the loss of what never came to be. It's not unusual to be consumed with regret from all of the missed opportunities and time spent in the unfruitful and unpleasant pursuit of shrinking your body.

There are five classic stages of grieving, which were identified and described by the pioneering work of psychiatrist Elisabeth Kübler-Ross.[31] While these stages originated from her work *On Death and Dying*, they can generally be applied to any loss. Here are the stages of grief and how they apply to diet culture:

- *Denial*: Disbelief that dieting doesn't work. Or thinking, "Not me, I'll be the exception."

- *Anger*: Outrage that dieting doesn't work. Anger at our culture for perpetuating fat phobia.

- *Bargaining*: The what-ifs, woulda-coulda-shouldas, and regrets. *What if I just go on one more diet? What if I lose weight first, then become an Intuitive Eater?*

- *Depression*: Sadness from the loss of time, loss of money, distraction from your life, and emotional energy spent in diet culture. Regret about how diet culture behavior interfered with the quality of your relationships. Feeling disappointment that dieting is no longer a viable coping mechanism or fantasy.

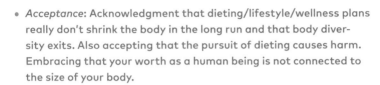

- *Acceptance*: Acknowledgment that dieting/lifestyle/wellness plans really don't shrink the body in the long run and that body diversity exits. Also accepting that the pursuit of dieting causes harm. Embracing that your worth as a human being is not connected to the size of your body.

There is no prescriptive or chronological timeline for the grieving process—this merely offers a framework, which describes the general stages of loss. You may even find yourself occupying several categories at once. Where do you fall in the stages of grief today?

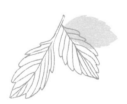

Day 271
Notice Relief from Body Shaming

How are you doing at letting go of body-shaming media? Is it surprising how pervasive this is? Are there any accounts that you are having trouble unfollowing? This is not unusual, because you may have developed a social connection or bond with the particular media outlet or influencer. There might be qualities of the account/show/person that you really like. If they were 100 percent jerks, it would be much easier to let go. As you leave behind these outlets, are you noticing any relief or shift of your own internalized body-shame dialogue?

Day 272

MEAL MEDITATIONS
Avoiding Performative Eating

May I stay attuned and true to my body's unique nourishment needs.
I shall not engage in performative eating, in which
I eat only to meet the expectations and approval of others.
I shall remember that only I know:
My true hungers and
What truly satisfies my personal tastes and appetite.
May I eat without judgment toward others or myself.

SELF-CARE
Schedule a Mental Health Day

It's important to give your mind a break from all the "shoulds" on your perpetual to-do list. Perhaps you've had days where you "got nothing done," and the stress of crossing something off your list was still hanging over your head. Behaviorally, you didn't complete your tasks, but mentally, there was no break or relief. That's why you can feel drained after doing nothing—you were up against the mental energy of a back-and-forth mental fight of "I should." The internal tug-o-war is exhausting.

Peace and power from within come from truly granting yourself permission, telling yourself, "I give myself permission to take a complete break," with no expectations or hidden agenda.

What would it be like to have a day where nothing is scheduled? Maybe you would sleep in. Maybe you would get up early to seize the day of relaxation. Maybe you would take a nap. Maybe you would spontaneously call a friend to get together for coffee and conversation. Perhaps you would take a relaxing walk. The day could be completely up to you! (If you are a parent with small kids, someone who is working full-time and going to school, or working multiple jobs to survive—you might not have the privilege of having an entire day to yourself. What might be a workable alternative?)

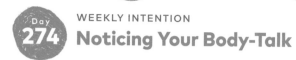

WEEKLY INTENTION
Noticing Your Body-Talk

Your body is your home for the rest of your life. It is the keeper of your values, character strengths, consciousness, and so forth. Living in a home fraught with hostility and loathing can make it difficult to tune in and self-connect.

Showing body respect includes paying attention to your thoughts and how you talk to yourself, which plays an important role in cultivating self-dignity.

This week: Notice your self-talk about your body. What is the frequency of this inner dialogue, and how often is it critical or denigrating? Even if a thought is true, does getting all caught up in it help you move in the direction of having a better relationship with your body?

Try replacing negative self-talk with kind self-talk, such as

- I am more than a body.

- All bodies are worthy of dignity and respect, including my own.

- My body does not define who I am or what I value.

Day 275

Grounding: Notice and Narrate

Grounding activities help you connect to the present moment. They usually involve perceiving your senses, because you can only access those in the here-and-now. Similarly, you can only access interoceptive awareness in the present moment. Working on awareness of your senses is a great practice to help you get ready to access interoceptive awareness.

PRACTICE

You can engage in this practice just about anytime, anywhere. Silently narrate what you *see*, *hear*, or *smell* in your current surroundings. Do this without trying to be clever or original. The process might go like this: I hear a siren in the distance, I see a large tree, and I smell pasta cooking.

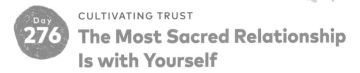

Day 276

The Most Sacred Relationship Is with Yourself

Self-trust is an integral component of your most sacred relationship, which is with yourself. Trust in yourself is a gateway to authentic connection with others. In order to connect with others, you need to be able to self-connect, which takes listening and self-trust. But diet culture slowly erodes and undermines this trust.

Please know that no matter how long you have been engaged in diet culture, it is possible to heal. Healing takes time, and that's okay. Your situation is workable. You can come home to yourself, your body, your wants, and your needs. Nobody could possibly know what those are, except for you. It's time to tend and befriend your body. It is never too late.

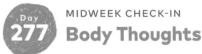

Day 277

Body Thoughts

Awareness of negative body talk can be daunting. And it's probably even more prevalent than you realize. If half of your waking hours are spent having negative thoughts about your body, that's a lot of body bashing, and negative thinking. That's why, in the beginning, reframing negative body thoughts may not seem to have an impact. First comes awareness, and then the practice of reframing with kind self-talk.

Day 278

INTUITIVE EATING MANTRAS

It's okay to go at my own pace—Intuitive Eating isn't a race.

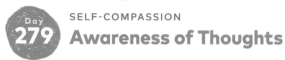

Day 279 Awareness of Thoughts

How often have you been completely unaware of your thoughts or behaviors until way after the fact? You are not alone. Consider that the majority of people spend close to 47 percent of their waking hours mind wandering, disconnected from the present moment.[32]

Only through awareness can meaningful change take place. In the learning process, this usually means you will need to pay attention to thoughts or actions that you don't like or would rather not experience. Becoming aware of destructive or unpleasant thoughts and actions as they arise in the moment is progress, even if it doesn't feel like it right then. Self-compassion will help you access this awareness sooner, because it's easier to look at your thoughts and behaviors through the lens of understanding kindness.

EMBODIED AFFIRMATIONS

Day 280

I Have Unconditional Positive Regard for Myself

Unconditional positive self-regard means accepting your humanity, as you are, without conditions.[33] Cultivating this internal acceptance allows you to connect to your inner resources and wisdom. Notably, this is the opposite of what diet culture does, which conditions you to place emphasis on external rules and standards.

PRACTICE

Reflect on a time when you had a sense of awe or love for your very essence of being human. Perhaps it was during a spiritual practice. Maybe it was when you were very young, and you saw the love from an important person in your life reflected back at you through their eyes—you felt it about yourself. When this situation is clear in your mind, connect with the feeling of this knowing awareness.

To amplify this feeling place your hand on your heart or in a self-hug, and slowly repeat three times, *"I have unconditional positive regard for myself."*

WEEKLY INTENTION

Take Inventory of Clothing and Undergarments

It can be quite aggravating and triggering to wear clothes that don't fit your here-and-now body comfortably. The operative word here is *comfortable*. Sure, you can squeeze into a pair of jeans, but if they are pinching you every time you sit or walk, they're really not fitting comfortably. Opening up your closet and truly not knowing what to wear because nothing seems to fit right is a hard way to start the day.

This week: Take inventory of your clothing, including undergarments. Evaluate your closet and dresser drawers to see if your clothing actually *feels* comfortable on your body. This also includes styles that you no longer like or wear. Bag up the clothing that does not feel right on your body. You don't need to give them away, unless you feel ready for that step. Put this clothing aside—under your bed or in your garage or some other out-of-the-way place.

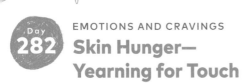

Day 282

Skin Hunger—Yearning for Touch

People living alone around the world collectively felt skin hunger from being deprived of touch during the COVID-19 pandemic. We are wired for touch; without it we wither.

The power of touch makes us feel calmer, happier, and safer. Fascinating research has shown that touch conveys an array of health benefits including[34]

- Stimulating the vagus nerve, which calms the nervous system and helps us feel safe;
- Lowering blood pressure and heart rate;
- Lowering cortisol, a stress hormone;
- Releasing oxytocin, the bonding hormone that helps us feel connected.

Fortunately, it's possible to get these benefits from self-touch, like putting lotion on your skin, washing your hair, and self-massage. Even stretching triggers the skin receptors that convey these health benefits.

If you find you have an unquenchable food craving that eating does not satisfy, it might be because the underlying need is skin hunger. Please remember, however, that there is no shame in self-soothing with food.

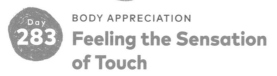

BODY APPRECIATION
Feeling the Sensation of Touch

Consider your everyday activities that involve touch, such as enjoying the sensation of water caressing your scalp during a shower, feeling the tickle of foamy soft soap on your hands as you wash the dishes, petting a friendly fluffy dog, or brushing your hair. If you didn't have a body, you would not be able to perceive these sensations. What do you appreciate about the sensation of touch?

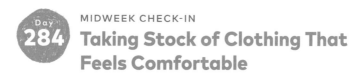

Day 284

MIDWEEK CHECK-IN
Taking Stock of Clothing That Feels Comfortable

How is your clothing inventory progressing? Perhaps you find yourself procrastinating. That's okay. Clothing is connected to so many events in life, both big and small. As a result, it can stir up a lot of emotions and memories. But remember, you have the right to wear clothing and undergarments that feel comfortable on your here-and now body. So please gently return to the importance of your clothing inventory, as you feel ready.

If you managed to make your way through most of your clothing, what is left that actually feels good on your body? Is it enough to get you through a week?

If your current clothing feels comfortable on your body, that's an awesome discovery too. Did you bag up any clothes that you no longer wear?

INTUITIVE EATING MANTRAS

Letting go of perfection
helps me to connect
with the process of
Intuitive Eating.

INTEROCEPTIVE AWARENESS

Grounding: Write Your Name, Age, and Capability

Sometimes it can be easy to get triggered and return to a time and place when you were younger, vulnerable, and feeling helpless. You need to feel safe in order to be present and access interoceptive awareness. This grounding activity will help remind you of your agency. To help ground you in the present moment, try saying to yourself or writing or typing into a phone, tablet, or computer

My name is _____.

I am an adult, _____ years old.

I can take care of my needs and myself. If I choose, I can _____ (choose of any of the following that apply to you):

- Drive a car out of here.

- Use a ride-sharing app out of here.

- Walk away from a situation.

- Buy my own food.

- Get out of town.

- Choose my friends and relationships.

- Find and use resources for solutions to my problems.

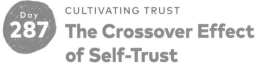

The Crossover Effect of Self-Trust

Day 287

Learning to trust your body activates a fascinating, empowering process: You begin trusting yourself in other parts of your life. At first you get little glimmers. Eventually, your entire self-trust is online and activated, rather than fragmented and discarded.

How could this be? Remember that your body is part of your internal navigation system. Embracing your body unconditionally aligns you with your inner knowing through the process of interoceptive awareness. Scientist A. D. Craig describes this as a global emotional moment—where the highest level of interoceptive integration represents the sentient self.[35]

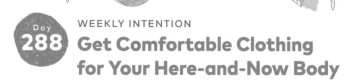

WEEKLY INTENTION

Day 288

Get Comfortable Clothing for Your Here-and-Now Body

When you have emptied your drawers and closets of clothing that does not fit comfortably or is out of style, you may find a gap in your clothing needs. It is incredibly helpful to acquire a few crucial pieces of clothing to fill out your wardrobe. The key is doing so while also honoring your financial constraints. This might mean saving up, shopping at a thrift store, organizing a clothing swap with friends, or asking for gift cards to your favorite clothing store, including online shops, for your next birthday gift.

This week: Keeping your finances in mind, make a plan to get a couple of basic articles of clothing that comfortably fit your here-and-now body—not your past body, not your wished-for future body. Consider starting with undergarments and build from there.

Day 289
Leaving Diet Culture Is Like Leaving an Abusive Relationship

The parallels are striking. In the beginning of an unhealthy relationship, the mistreated partner, might

- Rationalize that they just need to change their own behavior to make the relationship work, absolving the abusive partner of any wrongdoing. Similarly, dieters conclude that the solution is to try harder, again and again. *It will be different this time. Really!*

- Blame themselves for the relationship problems inflicted by the abuser. Likewise, dieters feel at fault, like failures. The multibillion-dollar dieting industry blames the consumer for "failed" dieting, rather than owning up to the truth that their product fails the consumer.

Progressively, the abused partner loses autonomy. Self-trust and confidence erode. When you finally get ready to leave the abusive relationship, you are showered with seductive empty promises to get you to stay or come back. Sound familiar?

The true culprit is our insidious diet culture that demonizes eating certain foods and normalizes body shame. Diet culture disconnects you from your body, your needs, and your life. It tells you what you can and cannot do. It demands obedience to and compliance with the rules. You are not the problem. Your body is not the problem. Diet culture is the problem and the abuser.

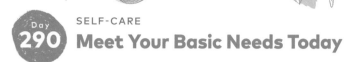

Day 290

Meet Your Basic Needs Today

How might you meet your needs today? Here are some ideas:

- Stay home when you are sick.

- Eat when you are hungry, rather than blow off a meal or snack.

- Reach out to others when you feel lonely or need help.

- Get enough sleep tonight by going to bed at a time that will give you the opportunity to do so.

- Say no to an event that will likely drain rather than renew you.

- Schedule your vacation time (and use it!).

- Take medication as prescribed.

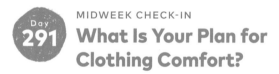

Day 291

MIDWEEK CHECK-IN

What Is Your Plan for Clothing Comfort?

It's okay to slowly create your plan to acquire clothing that fits your here-and-now body comfortably. Once it is complete, consider: What do you need to follow through with it? Maybe you need to be in the right place emotionally. Perhaps you need willingness and acceptance. Or maybe you need to consider your financial circumstances. Consider all these factors as you determine your next step.

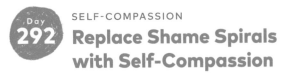

SELF-COMPASSION

Replace Shame Spirals with Self-Compassion

Shame is a self-denigrating emotion, the root of which is the belief that you are fundamentally unworthy and flawed. The emotion is fused with the idea that *you* are the flaw or the mistake, rather than the behavior you hope to change. Like a relentless whirlpool, the toilet vortex of self-shaming is a fast way to get sucked into negativity. It might start with something like this:

- "I'm damaged goods."

- "I'm f*cked up."

- "I'm the worst."

Self-compassion is the anecdote to shame. This means accepting the reality that humans make mistakes, but *you* are not a mistake. Accepting this truth with a tender kindness toward yourself eases suffering. It's possible to feel disappointed in your behavior, or the thought process that got you there, without destroying regard for your inner humanity. It's also possible to endure painful experiences without personalizing them.

Cultivating an open stance of nonjudgmental awareness will help you acknowledge your thoughts and feelings, without overidentifying with or denying them. The process might sound like this:

- "I am growing and learning from my mistakes. No one is perfect."

- "I am not my thoughts or my feelings."

- "A lot of people are struggling with their relationship with their body. I am working to find a way to heal, and it will take time to learn a kinder way to talk to myself and my body."

Day
293

INTUITIVE EATING MANTRAS

Making peace with
food and my
body is possible.

MEAL MEDITATIONS

Appreciating the Interconnectedness and Privilege of Receiving Food

May I recognize my privilege to buy food that nourishes my body.
May I honor the interconnected web of growing,
storing, and distributing food.
May I appreciate the farmer, fieldworker, truck
driver, grocery clerk, and all involved.
May I appreciate the interdependence of getting food on my plate.

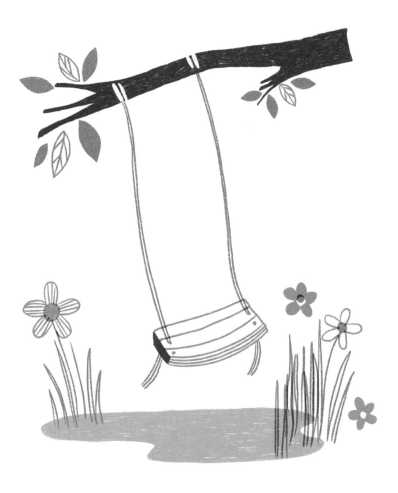

Movement—Feel the Difference

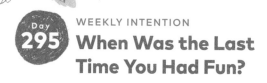

When Was the Last Time You Had Fun?

Just as Intuitive Eating helps you reclaim satisfaction in eating, it helps you reclaim joy in movement. Imagine moving your body without an agenda or compulsion—no worries about the duration, intensity, or calories burned. Seeking an activity for enjoyment can change your relationship to movement, especially if it's been fraught or connected to painful memories, such as teasing or punishments.

When was the last time you played or had fun moving your body? If that's hard to conjure—reflect on your childhood: Were there any games or activities you enjoyed as a kid (perhaps swimming, dancing, jumping rope)? Do any of those activities appeal to you now as an adult?

This week: Explore the possibility of trying one new activity based on enjoyment. The sky's the limit here! Consider games such as ping-pong, Hula-Hooping, Frisbee, handball, dodgeball, pickleball, or basketball. Contemplate activities that you might enjoy with your family or friends like roller-skating, playing catch, riding a bike, or walking and talking. Need some more inspiration? Check out Meetup.com for some ideas that don't require any commitment, fees, or equipment.

If your body is in pain or has conditions that make movement difficult, it's especially important to consider activities conducive to people of all sizes, abilities, and interests. This can include activities in a chair, such as chair yoga, chair tai chi, or Zumba chair dancing.

EMBODIED AFFIRMATIONS

I Am Not Responsible for Other People's Feelings

While you are certainly responsible for your words and actions toward others, you are not responsible for the feelings of other people. You cannot control people's reactions to your decisions; whether they deal with them rationally or not, understandingly or not, is up to them. If you make decisions based on the expected responses of other people, you are not living authentically, which can create a sense of unbalanced living.

If someone takes pride in making a special dish, for example, you are under no obligation to eat it in order to make them happy. You can certainly express appreciation or ask to take some home with you.

PRACTICE

Recall a time when someone was pushing food on you and expressed disappointment when you didn't eat it. Perhaps you were full or just had no interest in eating it. Notice the bodily relief in your decision of honoring your boundaries and amplify this feeling.

Put your hand on your heart or in a self-hug and slowly repeat three times, *"I am not responsible for other people's feelings."*

Day 297

LOVING BOUNDARIES

The Body Is Not a Punch Line

Fat phobia is not funny—it's a prejudice that harms people while perpetuating body shame and weight stigma. It also makes it hard for people recovering from eating disorders, disordered eating, and diet culture. Yet it is common for people to silently go along with fat jokes because they don't know what else to do or say. The problem is that silence is a form of complicity.

You can set boundaries in your spheres of influence, which include family, friends, coworkers, and other people you see regularly. You can speak up and let them know how this type of humor makes you feel. Here are some things you might say and actions you can take:

- I don't think fat jokes are funny.

- Insulting people's bodies is not funny.

- These jokes make me feel uncomfortable.

- It is unkind to make fun of people's bodies.

- People's bodies are not punch lines.

- Body objectification and jokes are the breeding ground for body image problems and eating disorders.

- Use your body language. Raise your hand in the air, gesturing, *Stop!* Follow up with something like, "I hope you are not about to tell a body-shaming joke. They are not funny and hurt people."

- Leave the conversation. While this does not set a boundary, it removes you from participating in toxic jokes and conversations.

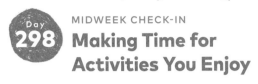

Day 298

Making Time for Activities You Enjoy

It's easier to make time for activities that you enjoy rather than dread. This may involve trying out several different types of activities to see what is really a match for you—like test-driving a car. It's important to have patience and take the time to figure out what really brings you joy.

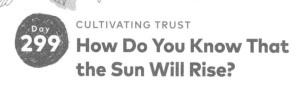

Day 299
How Do You Know That the Sun Will Rise?

Whether covered in clouds, rain, or snow, the sun rises every day. I have yet to meet a person who doesn't trust that this is true. How is it that we each possess a knowingness of this brilliant pattern of daily arising? We bloom and awaken with this cyclic knowledge, often taking it for granted. When we repeatedly witness this physical truth, we are conditioned to just *know*. Similarly, if you grew up with the repeated experiences and messages that your body is worthy of trust, you just *know* it to be true.

As soon as diet culture enters the scene, self-doubts start to emerge. Diet culture can manifest in the form of endless body and food comments by parents, teachers, coaches, family, friends, health-care professionals, wellness influencers, and media *ad infinitum*. Add to this years spent on diets and food plans to shrink your body, and you have a confluence of body doubt. It's understandable if you don't trust your body right now. This takes repeated, consistent experiences of treating your body kindly and nourishing it in a timely manner. With patience and practice, you will come to know and trust your body again.

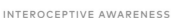

INTEROCEPTIVE AWARENESS

Day 300 Grounding: Feel an Ice Cube

Get an ice cube, and hold it in your hand.[36] (If holding an ice cube feels too intense, you can wrap the ice cube in a paper towel.) How does your hand react to the temperature of the ice? What sensations do you feel? Is the sensation isolated to just your hand, or does it seem to travel? Notice the color of your hand holding the ice—what do you see?

Day 301

INTUITIVE EATING MANTRAS

Pursuing intentional weight loss interferes with the process of Intuitive Eating.

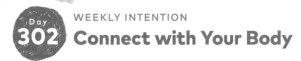

Day 302

Connect with Your Body

Moving your body for enjoyment is a unique opportunity to connect with it, which helps to strengthen interoceptive awareness. Every time you check in with the experience of your body, you are deepening the connection. This process takes time, practice, and patience.

This week: Notice how you feel while you are moving—whether it's stretching, balancing, walking, or dancing. How does this activity feel for your body: pleasant, unpleasant, or neutral? If you feel pleasant or neutral—awesome—take it one step further, get curious and notice what is contributing to this state. Perhaps you are wearing comfortable clothing. Maybe it's the right intensity or timing.

If you notice that you feel unpleasant, get curious as to why might that be—too much intensity, too much, too soon? Perhaps you feel an emerging injury? Maybe it's too hot? Perhaps you don't feel safe? There's no wrong or right answer. Just check in. What might you try next time for a more enjoyable experience?

Day 303
Feeling the "Need" for a New Body?

If you find that you are yearning for a new body, consider if the following might be true for you instead. Underneath the yearning, might you be feeling a desire for_____?

- Connection

- Community

- Acceptance

- Stamina

- Strength

- Belonging

- Autonomy

- Freedom

How could you work toward any of these qualities without putting the focus on changing your body?

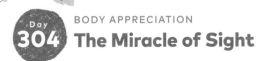

BODY APPRECIATION
The Miracle of Sight

Reflect on all the things you will be doing today—how many of them rely on eyesight? From the mundane to the surreal, whether it's navigating the road you travel or locking eyes with your lover—our vision is a powerful portal. It's the only part of our nervous system that is exposed to the outside world.

Thank you, eyes, for being a powerful connection with others. My eyes greet people and bear compassionate witness to their lives. My eyes express a variety of feelings from weeping a salty river of sorrow to tears of ebullient laughter. My eyes dazzle my soul upon viewing nature's striking vistas, evocative artistry from a painter's brush, or reading poetic offerings. In everyday life, my eyes help me watch a movie or video, read the news, or find my lost keys. My eyes are the witness of my life unfolding and guide me.

What do you appreciate about your eyes?

Day 305

Feeling the Connection with Your Body When Moving It

What have you noticed about the physical sensations of movement? Fixating on calories burned when you exercise keeps you externally focused, which disconnects you from your body. Paying attention to how you feel, by contrast, can prevent injuries and burnout while boosting enjoyment and fun. It also is a form of cross-training for Intuitive Eating, because this type of body awareness helps you notice sensations of hunger and fullness. It's all about internal awareness of sensation. And, with practice, this becomes clearer and easier.

SELF-CARE

Day 306

Know Thyself and Your Limits

Only you can be the expert of you. Only you know your thoughts, feelings, experiences, and emotional and energetic capacities. However, it's all too easy to get caught up in pleasing others and becoming completely others-focused. When you know your own limits and what you can realistically handle, setting boundaries to protect your essential self-care feels more natural. Setting and maintaining boundaries is an important skill set in assuring your self-care needs.

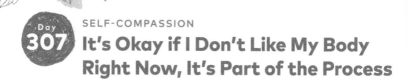

Day 307 It's Okay if I Don't Like My Body Right Now, It's Part of the Process

Do you believe that in order to become an Intuitive Eater you are required to like, accept, or love your body? It would be awesome if you truly felt that way, but it's vitally important that you are emotionally honest with your feelings.

Frankly, if you have been loathing your body for a good part of your life, it's not realistic to suddenly shift into liking your body. It's really understandable for anybody raised in diet culture to have internalized the thin ideal and fat phobia. There are people all over the world who feel this way.

It is completely possible to hold two conflicting mindsets—to be at war with your body while simultaneously wanting to truly feel at peace with it. As you shift your focus to valuing your person-hood and your humanity, rather than objectifying the skin you are in, your authentic feelings and kindness toward yourself will also shift.

Day 308

INTUITIVE EATING MANTRAS

By practicing Intuitive Eating, I am repairing my guilt-ridden relationship with food and body.

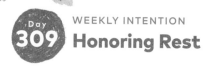

WEEKLY INTENTION
Honoring Rest

When you are caught in the throes of diet culture, physical activity can feel like a punishing obligation and compulsion. That's not good for your physical or mental health. It's important to be able to take time off and rest your body, especially if you are getting sick or feeling an emerging injury. The truth is that you will not lose fitness from missing a day or two, or even having a week of rest. Taking time off also helps to prevent burnout.

This week: Pay attention to how your body is feeling. Plan to take at least one extra day of rest. Notice how that idea makes you feel. Perhaps it triggers fear of losing your physical fitness or fears that you will not want to ever exercise again (a common fear when you have been relentlessly pushing your body). When you take that day off, notice how you feel the next time you move your body.

EMBODIED AFFIRMATIONS

Day 310
I Deserve to Be Happy in My Here-and-Now Body

How often have you postponed events and decisions until you were in the "right body"? Consider things like dating, going on a vacation, applying for a new job, learning a new sport, having children, and getting clothes that fit comfortably and are consistent with your style. This is not living. This is cultural conditioning and fat phobia.

This affirmation will help remind you that life is happening now and that you deserve to be happy, regardless of diet culture's noxious conditioning.

PRACTICE

Recall a time when you wholly participated in an event, regardless of how you were feeling in your body, and it was a positive experience. Perhaps the experience even surprised you! Perhaps it was when you went to a class reunion, the beach, a wedding, a date, or a vacation. When this event is firmly recollected in your mind, connect with the feeling of happiness, or contentment, or another positive emotion. Amplify this feeling.

Place your hand on your heart or in a self-hug and slowly repeat three times, *"I deserve to be happy in my here-and-now body."*

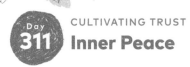

Day 311

Inner Peace

As you repair trust and connection with your body, there is an unfolding and a transcendence that results in a beautiful gift: a deep inner peace and knowingness. No one can take that away from you. Diet culture can yell loudly, waving its newest latest and greatest superfood, superplan, super-shrink-your-body-but-it's-not-a-diet rhetoric. You will not be drawn in, because you know your truth. Your body experience is your own. You become unshakeable in your knowing. It's not about feeling perfect about your body or your eating. Rather, it's staying rooted in your truth and not reacting or internalizing diet culture's endless barbs.

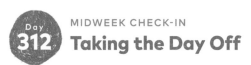

MIDWEEK CHECK-IN

Day 312

Taking the Day Off

Have you planned your extra day off from activity? This is also a good practice in cognitive flexibility—so you can honor the needs of your body. Sometimes, that need is rest. Rest can feel very difficult for some people. Our grind culture rewards and conditions us to be on the go, go, go—often at the expense of getting your needs met. Your worth should not be tied up in your productivity—movement or otherwise.

INTEROCEPTIVE AWARENESS

Grounding: See Your Feet, Feel Your Feet

At this moment, find a place to sit down—such as on a chair, couch, stool, or bench—with your feet on the floor. When you feel comfortable and settled in, take a couple of relaxing breaths. Now, place your awareness on your feet. Can you feel your soles touching the ground? What does the sensation feel like? Is there any sensation of hot, cold, or temperate? How do the tops of your feet feel? Wiggle your toes. How do your toes feel? How does the tissue inside your feet and toes feel? Do you have any aches, pains, pinches, numbness, tingling, or burning sensations?

Whether you are sitting or standing, when you connect with and feel your feet on the ground, you are present in the here and now. It can also be a powerful reminder—that I am rooted, I am breathing, and I am alive.

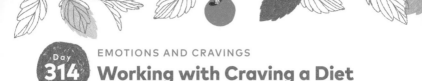

Day 314
Working with Craving a Diet

If you find yourself craving being on a diet *just one more time*, please know this is common. This desire actually provides an opportunity to look deeper. It's likely that when a craving for a diet, a.k.a. lifestyle change, presents itself there could be an unmet need or underlying emotion. When this occurs, explore these possibilities:

- *Am I yearning for certainty?* Diet culture and dieting offer a false promise of certainty.

- *Am I craving distraction from anxiety?* Diet culture offers profound distraction, such as from a new job, new school, or new life change.

- *Am I looking for excitement?* Diet culture offers excitement and fantasy.

- *Am I looking to fit in or belong?* Diet culture offers the fantasy of belonging via achieving an idealized body size and sharing a common goal of body alteration.

Consider other ways to meet these desires or needs without putting your mind and body in harm's way by reengaging with diet culture.

Day
315

INTUITIVE EATING MANTRAS

As air is essential to life, so is nourishment essential for my body.

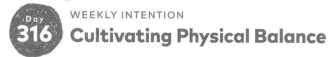

WEEKLY INTENTION
Cultivating Physical Balance

The ability to balance is a function of proprioception, which is our body's ability to know where we are in space at any given moment. Balance is something we often take for granted. Yet it is so important in everyday life—like for walking, sitting, and helping prevent injuries from falls and missteps. As you age, balance is an ability that declines. Fortunately, balance or proprioception can be cultivated.

This week: Consider trying any of these activities—which will help develop and preserve balance—that sound appealing to you: yoga, tai chi, barre, Pilates, martial arts, or basic balancing activities such as standing on one foot.

Day 317
Belonging: Connecting in a Different Way

True belonging is about living authentically in your truth, rather than trying to conform to the expectations of others. Once your eyes have been opened to the futility and harm of diet culture, you just can't unsee it. You just can't participate in it any longer. It's common to go through a period of unease and grieving as you disconnect from the tentacles of diet culture. This is to be expected. There is nothing wrong with you. It's a transition and a paradigm shift.

During this season, it can be helpful to begin exploring ways to connect with a new community, or activities that support and renew you. You can try very simple things like gardening, joining a book club, joining a volunteer organization, participating in an online support group, or curating your social media feed with positive, inspiring accounts free from diet culture.

Day 318

MEAL MEDITATIONS
Self-Connection

May I be connected to the sensations of eating.
May I delight in the sight, taste, aroma, sound,
and textures of my meal.
May I appreciate that with each bite, I am healing my
relationship and connection with food.
May I value that each time I honor hunger, I am rebuilding
trust and connection with my body.

Day 319

MIDWEEK CHECK-IN
Balancing Act

Have you tried any activities to improve your balance? How would improved balance impact your quality of life? If you would like an easy assessment of your balance, try this activity. With a wall or support nearby, see if you can stand on one leg for thirty seconds or more without swaying or losing your balance. Remember, this has no bearing on your value as a person—please approach this practice with gentle curiosity and exploration!

SELF-COMPASSION

No Matter What You Ate Yesterday, Your Body Still Needs Nourishing Today

It's important to let go of yesterday. Diet culture conditions you to compensate for any perceived eating indiscretions. Consequently, you might notice a panicky reactivity to restrict your eating if you thought you ate too much. But doing that disconnects you from your body. It reinforces the notion of living by the rules in your head, instead of by the direct experiences of your here-and-now body. Compensating for perceived eating mistakes robs you of the experience of seeing how your body would adjust naturally, if needed, which further erodes trust in your body.

It's understandable that you have a habit of thinking to cut back on your eating. What is a kind way you can let go of yesterday (or even this morning) and take care of your body in the present moment?

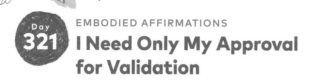

EMBODIED AFFIRMATIONS

Day 321
I Need Only My Approval for Validation

Culture conditions us to conform and obey. Over time, you start to lose yourself and look toward others for approval. This affirmation will remind you of your own authority and agency.

PRACTICE

Recall a time when you took an action for yourself that worked out really well. Perhaps it was when you went on a spiritual journey different from your upbringing, went back to school, changed careers, spoke your truth, or made an unpopular decision. This doesn't need to be a big event or decision—even a glimmer will do. When this decision or event is firmly recollected in your mind, connect with the feeling of self-knowing. Now amplify that feeling.

Place your hand on your heart or in a self-hug and slowly repeat three times, *"I need only my approval for validation."*

CULTIVATING TRUST

Expectations of Perfectionism Erode Trust

No one is born perfect. There is no such thing as perfect eating, perfect thinking, a perfect body, or a perfect life. Even our DNA, our vital life code, mutates! When you strive for perfection, you go against nature. There's nothing wrong with having aspirations or doing your best. But having an expectation of perfection turns life into a performance, and it comes at a big price. You lose your authenticity and connection to your true self. This gradually morphs into self-doubt; you might even feel like you don't know who you are.

When you've been caught up in the pursuit of "perfect" eating, according to the latest and greatest diet fad, you will likely find yourself getting to a point of feeling like you "don't know how to eat anymore" (even if you have a lot of food and nutrition knowledge). This will change as you start shifting and prioritizing your focus to connecting with your body and how it feels.

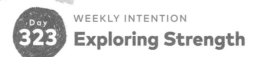

Day 323

WEEKLY INTENTION
Exploring Strength

Strength is a component of movement to explore because it impacts our quality of life. For example, just a single bout of strength training has been shown to help with anxiety.[37] It can prevent injuries, help your muscles and bones get stronger, improve blood pressure and mood, help regulate your blood sugar, and slow the natural loss of muscle that occurs with aging. Strength training is also known as resistance training, which means you can use your own body weight (like in yoga) or use bands to build strength.

This week: Explore fun ways you can incorporate strength-building activities into your life. Consider checking out these YouTube videos (most are less than 30 minutes) for ideas:

- "Yoga for Beginners: Getting Back to Your Mat Part 1" (Dianne Bondy Yoga)

- "Handless Vinyasa for Lower Body Strength and Balance" (Dianne Bondy Yoga)

- "Gentle Yoga for Bigger Bodies" (The Yoga Room)

- "30-Minute Strength & Conditioning Workout with Warm Up & Cool Down" (Self, no equipment)

- "Total Body Resistance Bands Workout" (JJ Dancer)

- "Senior Fitness—Resistance Band Exercises Full Body Workout" (Senior Fitness with Meredith)

- Seated Upper Body Exercise Video | Kaiser Permanente (Kaiser Permanente Thrive, under 50 minutes)

Day
324

INTUITIVE EATING MANTRAS

Intuitive Eating is a healthy resistance against diet culture and weight stigma.

LOVING BOUNDARIES

Concern Trolling: I'm Concerned About Your Health

Concern trolling as it pertains to diet culture is a sanitized form of fat phobia carried out under the guise of "concerns about health." On the surface, it appears to be a socially acceptable way to comment on someone's body size: "I'm just concerned about your health."

Contrary to popular belief, you cannot discern a person's health by looking at the size of their body. The same holds true for identifying eating disorders, athletic abilities, and character traits. Major confounding factors play a key role in health—but they are not factored in the often-biased lens of "weight science." These factors include, but are not limited to, Adverse Childhood Experiences (ACEs), social isolation, loneliness, sleep deprivation, trauma, social determinants of health, poverty, racism, weight cycling, and weight stigma.

Whether the concern is well-meaning or mean-spirited, it's not acceptable to comment on someone else's body. Here are some things you can say:

- Please don't comment on my body or my health.

- It's my body and my personal business.

- My body is not up for discussion.

- The problem is fat phobia, not my body.

- My health is a personal matter between my health-care team and me.

- Making comments about my body, regardless of your intention, is not good for my health.

MIDWEEK CHECK-IN
Strengthening Opportunities

Have you discovered any strengthening exercises that look fun or interesting to you? It's important to match the activity with where your body is and to begin slowly, when you feel ready. There is no rush here—let your body be your guide!

Day 327
INTEROCEPTIVE AWARENESS
Notice the Physical Sensation of Relief

Our descriptor language offers clues about the felt sense of relief, such as *"that's a weight off my shoulders"* or *"that's a load off my mind"* or *"a huge weight was lifted."* When you feel a burden being lifted or a load being lightened—whether it's getting your to-do list completed, finding out you passed the test, or getting the job—there's a felt sense in your body.

> **PRACTICE**
> The next time you experience some type of mental relief, notice the shift in your body. What does it feel like overall? Perhaps a lightness? Where do you feel it in your body?

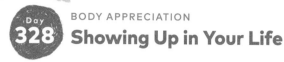

BODY APPRECIATION
Day **328** **Showing Up in Your Life**

Have you ever canceled plans because you feel uncomfortable in your body? As humans, we are wired to connect. Relationships have the power to nourish our mind and soul, and confer health benefits that add to our quality of life and longevity. Isolation heightens feelings of loneliness, anxiety, and depression.

PRACTICE

Set the intention to show up for a social event regardless of how you feel about your body. What would you need in order to follow through? Clothing that fits comfortably? Focusing on conversation, rather than distressing body thoughts?

Day 329

If You Are Seeking Health: Create Goals That Are Not Based on Weight

Some people mistakenly believe that taking the focus off weight means that you don't care about health. That's a huge misconception. Keep in mind that weight is not a behavior, nor is it an indicator of health or fitness. There is nothing wrong with wanting to feel healthy. Nor is health a moral imperative.

If you want to pursue healthy behaviors, there are many ways to do that without focusing on weight. Here are some ideas to contemplate:

- Get enough sleep, consistently.

- Move your body in ways that feel good.

- Cultivate and invest in meaningful relationships.

- Learn how to meditate.

Honor Health with Gentle Nutrition

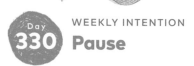

WEEKLY INTENTION
Pause

When you hear the word *nutrition* how does it make you feel? Does it send chills of anxiety down your spine? Perhaps it instills a sense of dread or shame? It's vitally important that your relationship with food, mind, and body feels mostly healed before you practice this principle. Unfortunately, diet culture has perpetuated shame about both food choices and body sizes. This is a form of trauma that needs to be healed. A growing body of research shows that shame has a profound impact on mental and physical health.[38]

While nutrition may play a role in preventing many chronic diseases, there are other factors that have an even more profound impact on your health:

- Social determinants of health, which include factors such as racism, economic status, access to health care, and where you live.

- Trauma or adverse childhood experiences. In the United States alone, at least five of the top ten leading causes of death are associated with adverse childhood experiences.

- Relationships and social connection. Loneliness and social isolation is considered one of the most profound public health problems.

There is absolutely no shame or judgment for choosing to delay working on this principle. Remember, mental health is just as important as physical health. Consider it a form of self-care to dive into this principle when you feel ready to proceed. Only you can determine when that will be.

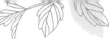
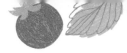

SELF-CARE

Evaluating Whether to Take on a New Project or Responsibility

It's all too easy to jump into projects and opportunities when it's something you really want to do. The key is to evaluate the possible consequences of saying yes. Here are some clarifying questions to help you assess impact:

- Is this opportunity aligned with my values and vision?

- Is it aligned with one of my needs—such as experiential, financial, or educational?

- Will this renew me, drain me, or have a neutral impact on my emotional energy?

- Do I have the time and energy? If not, is there another obligation I am willing (and able) to let go of in order to fully participate?

Sometimes the kind action, for both yourself and the other party, is to turn down the opportunity, especially if you really don't have the time to give it the attention it needs to be effective.

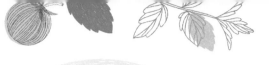

Day 332

INTUITIVE EATING MANTRAS

Intuitive Eating can help stop the legacy of diet culture in my family. It begins with me.

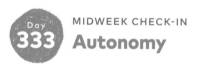

Day 333

MIDWEEK CHECK-IN
Autonomy

How does it feel to decide for yourself whether you are ready to work on the Honor Your Health with Gentle Nutrition principle? How does this feeling compare with someone telling you what to do? This is about autonomy and knowing your individual needs, ultimately deciding for yourself what is in your best interest. It's okay to pause and come back to this principle when *you* feel ready.

CULTIVATING TRUST

Micromanaging and Controlling Your Eating Disrupts Trust

When you attempt to control every bite of food that crosses your lips, you rob yourself of the opportunity to see how your body naturally regulates and guides your eating. In other words, micromanaging deprives you of the direct experience (and evidence) that your body works. After months or even years of this, it's understandable that you would have a lot of doubt and eroded trust.

The next time you perceive that you ate "too much" food or the "wrong" type of food, try noticing what happens with curious awareness, without micromanaging a corrective action. Kindly get out of your own way and let your body show you what it can do.

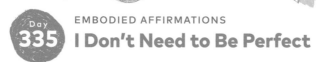

Day 335

EMBODIED AFFIRMATIONS

I Don't Need to Be Perfect

No one is infallible. Striving to live up to the impossible ideal of perfectionism keeps you stuck and perpetually anxious. This practice will affirm that making mistakes is part of the Intuitive Eating path—it's how you learn and grow.

PRACTICE

Recall a time when you learned something about yourself because you made a mistake. Maybe you went too long without eating and learned the power of primal hunger and biology. Perhaps you didn't listen to your body and worked out too hard or too much and got injured. When this situation is recollected in your mind, connect with the feeling of a knowing understanding.

Amplify this feeling, place your hand on your heart or in a self-hug, and slowly repeat three times, *"I don't need to be perfect."*

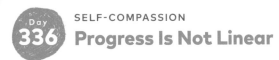

Day 336
Progress Is Not Linear

Even if you intellectually understand that progress is not linear, it is completely normal to feel stuck at times. It's actually part of the learning process.

Sometimes, we hold the unrealistic expectation of consistent progress. If you have spent years dieting or micromanaging your eating, it's just not realistic to expect a couple of months of hard work to liberate you from the diet culture mindset (let alone to learn the new language of listening to your body). Please know that there is value in steady, mundane self-connection, even if it seems like a plateau of nothing new.

This is an opportunity to practice self-compassion, especially if your tendency has been to berate yourself during tough times. Keep in mind that you cannot bully yourself into growth or into self-love. It's normal to feel frustrated and stuck at times—you are not alone.

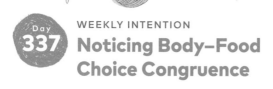

WEEKLY INTENTION
Noticing Body–Food Choice Congruence

Nourishment is so much more than the nutritional content of the foods we choose to eat. Agonizing over food decisions can wreak havoc on your mental health, adding unnecessary stress and suffering. It's fine to pursue healthy eating, as long as your relationship to food is also healthy.

Relying only on external indicators of nutrition shifts the focus away from the experience of your body, which includes taste and the effects of how food feels in your body—during and after eating. The latter is known as body–food choice congruence and is actually a form of interoceptive awareness, a very personal experience.

This week: Notice how food *feels* in your body during and after eating. For example, you may love a giant salad for lunch, and may feel great while eating it. But perhaps the salad doesn't feel sustaining—and you find yourself hungry just an hour or two later. Or perhaps you notice that you love the taste of donuts for breakfast, but you don't like how it feels in your body if you eat them solely as a meal. Or maybe you love the taste of chili and cornbread for dinner, and you enjoy the hearty feeling of the meal in your body. There's no wrong or right here; it's about your unique experience with eating.

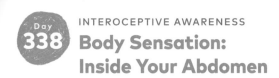

Day 338

Body Sensation: Inside Your Abdomen

A lot of our emotions are experienced in the abdomen. The more you can familiarize yourself with the sensations in this area, the more it will help you distinguish hunger cues from emotional sensations.

Trigger warning: Before starting this practice, please read through the entire process. If you feel uncomfortable with any aspect, or have a trauma history, please feel free to skip it. We are going to start this practice by having you notice surface sensations. Then, we'll move to the sensations within your body.

Take either a relaxed seated position, with your back firmly against a chair, or lie down on your back (on a bed, a mat, or the ground will be fine). First, notice the sensation of your back pressed against the chair or the ground.

Put one hand on your abdominal area. Place your awareness on the sensation between your hand and your skin. What do you notice? Keep your attention there until you can clearly detect the sensation of your hand on your abdomen.

Lastly, place your awareness inside your abdominal area, in the tissue in between the feeling of your back touching the surface and your hand. Notice the sensation you feel. Does it have a texture? A color? A shape? Overall, would you categorize the sensation as pleasant, unpleasant, or neutral?

Day 339

INTUITIVE EATING MANTRAS

My character and worth are not defined by my food choices.

MIDWEEK CHECK-IN

How Does Food Feel in Your Body After a Meal or Snack?

The more you notice body–food choice congruence, the more you begin to develop a personal catalogue of experiences, of true knowing. You will be able to predict what type of meal or snack is best for you—what feels good in your body and what sustains you. For example, you will have a better idea of what to eat in stressful situations, such as before giving a talk or going to a job interview. You want to be nourished and sustained, but you also don't want to feel uncomfortably full. This type of true knowing also helps heal your relationship with food, as you realize your body is worthy of your trust.

Day 341

MEAL MEDITATIONS

Nourishment Is Transformation

Just as the sun nourishes plants to grow and bloom,
Food turns into my body,
Into living cells, living tissue, living organs.
May I be in awe and appreciation of the transformation
of food into body!

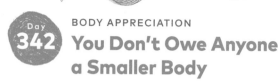

BODY APPRECIATION

You Don't Owe Anyone a Smaller Body

If you have a partner who pressures you to be a different size or to lose weight, that is not love. It's objectification. Our bodies change—they are supposed to. We are dynamic, living, ever-evolving beings. Healthy relationships are founded on love, mutual respect, and autonomy. Sometimes the body becomes the false argument that represents deeper conflicts in a relationship. It can feel much easier and safer to blame the physical body, rather than tackle the messy work of relationship issues.

If you don't have a partner and have put off the dating process until your body is the right size by societal standards, you are doing a disservice to yourself (reinforcing self-objectification and weight stigma). Having a partner who values your character and humanity, rather than valuing you just for your body, is critical for your mental health. People of all shapes and sizes find healthy, fulfilling love. You deserve this too, if it's something you desire.

LETTING GO OF DIET CULTURE

Teach Your Children Well— Stop the Legacy of Diet Culture

If you have children—or plan to—the idea that you can end the legacy of diet culture in your own family can be profoundly meaningful, healing, and empowering. You can help your children by preventing the unnecessary suffering caused by diet culture, which is often transmitted as a family value, generation by generation.

What this might mean:

- Tell extended family members that you don't want to expose your kids to diet talk, wellness talk, or body praise or criticism. They don't have to agree with your reasons—they just need to respect your boundary.

- Keep in mind that you are not asking anyone to change their own eating behaviors and activity patterns—because you believe in body autonomy. Rather, you are asking them not to discuss or gossip about these issues around your kids.

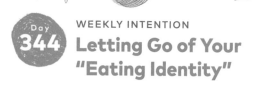

WEEKLY INTENTION
Letting Go of Your "Eating Identity"

Sometimes, a special way of eating gives a person an identity, which makes them feel unique and even superior to other people. But this is really a hard way to live and when rigidly adhered to can contribute to social isolation or an eating disorder.

It's truly fine to want to be healthy and feel good—but it isn't required for your humanity. You do not need to engage in performative eating, or actually be in good health, in order to have dignity or self-worth. Unfortunately, because of toxic diet culture, people in larger bodies may feel the need to eat this way in order to feel safe eating in public. Sadly, they are constantly being given unsolicited advice and even bullied about their eating by family, coworkers, friends, and complete strangers. (That's one of the reasons we need to work to dismantle diet culture.)

This week: Explore qualities and characteristics that you value about yourself that have nothing to do with how you eat. If this feels challenging, it may be helpful to imagine how a friend or a loved one would describe you. What would it be like to let go of your eating identity?

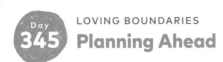

LOVING BOUNDARIES
Planning Ahead

If you want to improve your quality of life and lessen your stress load, it's much better to set boundaries in advance, rather than waiting until the moment of crisis when you need them. When your unstated boundaries are crossed, it's all too easy to become reactive or so caught off guard that you freeze and say nothing, while internally seething.

We can set boundaries to protect ourselves from diet culture. Setting and maintaining boundaries is an ongoing practice. Proactive boundaries can look like the following (perhaps over a phone call, email, or in-person conversation):

- When we get together for lunch, I would appreciate if we would not talk about or criticize anyone's food choices or dietary laments, including your own.

- I just want to let you know that if your neighbor cannot stop talking about her diet, I will quietly exit the conversation.

- I really need a body-shaming-free space. Can we establish this expectation before our next get-together?

- I'd rather not talk about anyone's diet at our next family gathering.

346 CULTIVATING TRUST
Context Changes Everything

What if you viewed your relationship with your body from the perspective of "It's understandable that I have self-doubt and mistrust of my body—it was culturally conditioned by my _____." (Insert what fits your situation here, such as family, friends, community, wellness influencers, diet culture, health-care providers, parents, body history, and/or dieting history.)

The most important realization with this perspective is that what has been culturally conditioned can also be unlearned and deconditioned. Imagine if each time you feel mistrusting of your body, you kindly remind yourself, "Ahh, that's my conditioning, and I'm working to unlearn it."

Day

347 MIDWEEK CHECK-IN
Letting Go of Performative Eating

Were you conditioned to believe that you have to perform in order to be loved or to prove your worth? The truth is that every human being is inherently worthy of dignity and respect, no performance required. This includes performative eating, such as being known as the "healthy one" or eating in a way to please the expectations of others. You might find that when you let go of that performance, it creates more mind space, which helps you connect authentically to yourself and others. What do you need in order to feel safe to let go of performative eating?

Day
348

INTUITIVE EATING MANTRAS

Intuitive Eating is my inner homecoming—it doesn't stop at the end of my fork. It's about connection and body dignity.

EMBODIED AFFIRMATIONS

My Lived Experience Is My Truth

Your valuable lived experiences are housed in your body and mind—the keepers of your truths. Diet culture undermines this sacred inner knowing. This practice affirms and recognizes your lived experience as an important part of cultivating a healthy relationship with food, mind, and body.

PRACTICE

Recall a time from your own experience when you had a realization that abiding by someone else's food rules or body ideal was harmful to you—your body and mind. You knew this from within your experience, perhaps feeling a deep knowingness. When this reflection is clear in your mind, connect with that feeling of inner knowing.

Amplify this feeling, place your hand on your heart or in a self-hug, and slowly repeat three times, *"My lived experience is my truth."*

EMOTIONS AND CRAVINGS
Losing Contact with Emotions

We learn to manage and regulate our emotions in childhood. But if you were shamed or taught that you are not allowed to have emotions, they become suppressed. Sometimes suppression is a way of surviving childhood and/or trauma. Children need a safe environment and caregivers who can help soothe and validate emotions. Without this practice of emotional regulation, you don't learn how to trust, let alone manage, turbulent emotional states. Sometimes experiencing emotions becomes a source of fear in and of itself—a fear of being hijacked by emotions.

Fortunately, healing is possible. There are new and effective therapies to work with these issues that are rooted in attachment, family systems, and trauma frameworks. You might need to work with a trusted therapist to help you with healing.

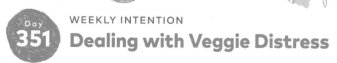

WEEKLY INTENTION
Dealing with Veggie Distress

When you've been steeped in diet culture, it's common to feel conflicted about eating veggies. Consider the following situations. Perhaps you feel

- Veggie averse—It's easy to develop a dislike of eating vegetables when you associate them with dieting and restrictive food plans. Consequently, it's usually a punitive and flavorless association.

- Fear that eating veggies will trigger dieting—It's common for new Intuitive Eaters to be reluctant to eat vegetables because they fear they will be headed down the rabbit hole of diet culture.

- Guilty for not eating enough—Sometimes people feel guilty if they aren't hitting a daily veggie quota.

Diet culture doesn't get to claim veggies. If you feel ready to explore reclaiming vegetables, keep reading. If not, by all means, skip this practice for now!

This practice is about shifting the focus to the enjoyment of eating veggies in a variety of forms, flavors, and textures. Nothing kills the joy of eating like a serving of guilt. Please remember, it's also important to consider your pattern of eating over a few days or weeks, rather than just one day.

This week: Notice how you feel during and after you eat veggies as a meal, a side dish, or garnish. Explore flavorful ways to include vegetables to your meals—perhaps explore new seasonings and spices, add nuts, or use a dipping sauce.

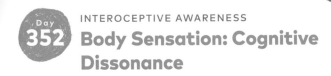

Day 352
Body Sensation: Cognitive Dissonance

Cognitive dissonance is a conflicting state in which your thoughts or actions, including speech, don't align with your beliefs. It is the discomfort you feel when holding conflicting ideas, beliefs, or values at the same time. It's a very unsettling feeling. Often, its presence will be felt first in your body. Something doesn't feel right—it feels off.

The pursuit of intentional weight loss is an example of something that creates cognitive dissonance with Intuitive Eating. A robust body of research shows that dieting does not work for the vast majority of people—it's not sustainable, increases your risk of gaining *more* weight than you lost (remember that weight gain is not inherently negative), and causes harm both biologically and psychologically.[39]

This is true whether your intention for shrinking your body is for "health" or appearance, whether you call it a "diet" or a "lifestyle," and whether you work with a health professional or not! In fact, the great majority of these studies showing harm and inefficacy have been under medical supervision.

Furthermore, pursuing weight loss interferes with the process of becoming an Intuitive Eater, because it shifts your focus to external rules of eating, rather than internal processes. Notice how the idea that diets don't work makes you feel. Does it make you mad? Does it put you in a state of cognitive dissonance? Where do you feel it in your body?

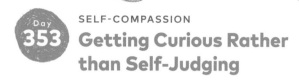

Day 353
Getting Curious Rather than Self-Judging

When you are exploring your body and food thoughts, practice invoking words of gentle curiosity rather than self-judgment:

I wonder what led to this _____

- Overpowering food-craving and subsequent binge?

- Total disregard of my biological hunger?

- Shame spiral about my body?

Is it possible that _____

- I had unrealistic expectations?

- I was triggered by a past trauma?

- I still have some healing to do?

Day 354
MIDWEEK CHECK-IN
The Joy of Eating

Remember that your body doesn't punch a time clock. You will not suddenly get a nutrient deficiency from one day or one week of eating. How are you doing with trying different flavorful ways to eat veggies?

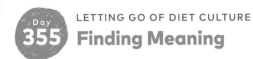

LETTING GO OF DIET CULTURE
Finding Meaning

One way to heal from and release diet culture is by perspective taking through finding meaning, which looks different for each person. We can't change the past, but we can learn from it. Deep learning (and unlearning) can help you transcend and let go.

Contemplate what you have learned about yourself through participating in diet culture and letting go by reflecting on these questions:

- Has it changed the way you view other people, other bodies?
- Has it given you a different perspective about how you want to raise your family?
- Has it shifted the way you interact with people?
- Has it clarified your values and/or passions?

Lastly, perhaps your own lived experience has taught you that dieting doesn't work, which will or does insulate you from diet culture's continual shape-shifting rhetoric.

Day 356

INTUITIVE EATING MANTRAS

There is no such thing as a perfect Intuitive Eater.

Day 357

SELF-CARE

Create a Musical Playlist for Self-Soothing and Relaxing

Music is powerful—it's a direct portal to our emotions and can even calm our nervous system.[40] Create and curate musical playlists for a variety of mood states with music that

- Soothes and relaxes;

- Energizes and helps you discharge restless energy;

- Connects with unexpressed feelings such as sadness or anger;

- Uplifts and transcends.

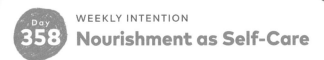

Day 358

Nourishment as Self-Care

Sometimes your hunger cues can be completely offline due to stress or illness. Your body still needs nourishment during these times. This is when you rely on your wise mind, in combination with your past experiences, to figure out kind ways to nourish your body. Part of the practice here is knowing what foods you like and tolerate, as well as what will sustain you. Another key issue is your energy level. For example, when you are sick, you will not likely have the energy to cook a three-course meal (even if you enjoy cooking). At times like this, it may be important to give yourself permission to take the night off from cooking. Maybe it means relying on some tried-and-true frozen meals or frozen leftovers. This is when it can be helpful to plan ahead, and the Nourishment as Self-Care Plan supports you in doing just that.

This week: Create Your Nourishment as Self-Care Plan by answering these questions (while keeping in mind affordability, storage, and cooking facilities that you have available):

Meals: What easy meals that taste good and will sustain you could you likely tolerate? Perhaps soup and toast? A grilled cheese sandwich? Something liquid like a smoothie?

Snacks: What are some easy snacks that you tolerate, that could fill in the gaps between meals? Consider these possibilities: yogurt, peanut butter on toast, banana and ice cream, cereal and milk, dried nuts and fruit, latte and fruit.

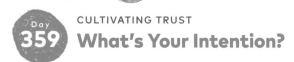

Day
359

What's Your Intention?

Sometimes, doing the very same behavior could either be an indication that you are slipping back into diet culture or an indication that you are prioritizing self-care—it all comes down to intention. It can be tricky to distinguish between the two and may create a wedge in your self-trust. For instance, perhaps you decide to meal prep for the week. Using meal prep to restrict your food intake is a diet culture behavior. On the other hand, using meal prep to save money and take the stress out of cooking, especially when you are short on time, is an awesome form of self-care. Another example is choosing an entrée salad for lunch. Eating salads to minimize food intake indicates diet culture behavior. If a salad sounds delicious and refreshing, however, that honors the satisfaction principle of Intuitive Eating.

A helpful question in times of uncertainty is *What is the intention behind my behavior?*

Keep in mind that there is no shame in discovering a lingering diet culture intention. If that's the case, thank yourself for your emotional honesty. That builds self-trust! Next, consider how you might tweak the behavior to support your Intuitive Eating journey.

Day 360

Engaging with Diet Culture and Social Justice Issues

Once you become aware of diet culture, you begin to see it everywhere. Dismantling diet culture takes energy, and if you are in this for the long haul (and I hope you are), it's vital that you protect your finite energy. Advocacy is important, and I believe we can change the culture one conversation at a time.

You are not required to engage with or educate every person who is determined not to "get it." To help discern how much time and energy to invest in a conversation, or whether to engage at all, I find it helpful to factor in my energetic bandwidth combined with the sage words from social justice advocate Desiree Adaway, "Are they reachable, teachable, and ready?"

MIDWEEK CHECK-IN

Day 361

Easy Access Nourishment as Self-Care

Consider an easily accessible place to store your Nourishment as Self-Care Plan, such as in a notes program on your cell phone or in an email to yourself. This will allow you to tweak and add to the list as you go about your life. Be sure you have some simple no-cook options such as picking up takeout or popping something into the microwave.

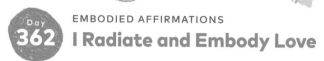

EMBODIED AFFIRMATIONS

I Radiate and Embody Love

Being raised and living in an appearance-based diet culture can instill a sense of not belonging, especially since the vast majority of people don't conform to the societally worshipped thin ideal. Over time, love for yourself and from others may feel conditional on your appearance. Not only are you loveable, at your core you are an emanation of love. This is true regardless of what you see in the mirror. This practice affirms your true essence of love.

PRACTICE

Recall a time when you felt love toward yourself. Perhaps it was when you were very young. Maybe when you were deep in nature and looking at a sunset or incredible vista and felt a loving connection toward yourself. Perhaps this feels like an extraordinarily difficult task. Sit with this for a while, and see if an event or situation arises. If not, reflect on a time when you felt deep love for a pet or another person. Connect with this loving feeling. Now amplify that feeling and direct it toward yourself.

Place your hand on your heart or in a self-hug, and slowly repeat three times, *"I radiate and embody love."*

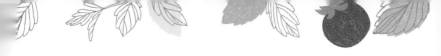

Day
363

INTUITIVE EATING MANTRAS

As I get more connected
to the wants and needs
of my mind and body, I
discover that the path
of Intuitive Eating is
life changing.

LETTING GO OF DIET CULTURE

Having Compassion for Those Stuck in Diet Culture

It is really common to get triggered or annoyed when hearing other people talk effusively about the latest diet lifestyle du jour. Remember when you used to feel like that—giddy with hope and excitement? Remember feeling convinced that you found the answer this time, really and truly? Eventually, and predictably, you got humbled into the belief that this diet lifestyle does not work and comes with a big price. Living in the throes of diet culture is an existence of suffering, preoccupation, and disappointment.

There will come a time when you are fully liberated from diet culture, and you will have genuine compassion for those who are still entangled in its web. People will change when and if they feel ready. Sometimes they need their own experiences and realizations to let go of diet culture. And when they do, you can help show them the way.

Day
365

MEAL MEDITATIONS

Appreciating Privilege

May there be an end to unnecessary suffering.
May no person go hungry.
May there be food security throughout the world.
May I not take for granted the privilege of eating this nourishing meal.

Practices and Inspirations Listed by Category

BODY APPRECIATION:
Days 5, 24, 44, 58, 77, 91, 107, 126, 146, 160, 175, 196, 213, 233, 248, 265, 283, 304, 328, 342

CULTIVATING TRUST:
Days 2, 14, 26, 38, 49, 61, 73, 86, 98, 110, 122, 133, 145, 156, 168, 180, 192, 205, 217, 229, 241, 252, 264, 276, 287, 299, 311, 322, 334, 346, 359

EMBODIED AFFIRMATIONS:
Days 13, 28, 41, 55, 69, 83, 97, 114, 128, 142, 157, 171, 184, 198, 212, 226, 240, 254, 266, 280, 296, 310, 321, 335, 349, 362

EMOTIONS AND CRAVINGS:
Days 16, 40, 65, 87, 112, 143, 188, 220, 257, 282, 314, 350

INTEROCEPTIVE AWARENESS:
Days: 3, 19, 33, 52, 66, 80, 96, 111, 125, 138, 152, 166, 181, 195, 209, 223, 237, 250, 262, 275, 286, 300, 313, 327, 338, 352

INTUITIVE EATING MANTRAS:
Days 9, 17, 27, 35, 42, 51, 59, 68, 76, 84, 94, 101, 108, 115, 124, 131, 139, 147, 154, 161, 170, 178, 185, 194, 202, 210, 219, 227, 236, 244, 251, 259, 268, 278, 285, 293, 301, 308, 315, 324, 332, 339, 348, 356, 363

LETTING GO OF DIET CULTURE:
Days 7, 20, 34, 48, 62, 75, 90, 104, 119, 135, 150, 164, 177, 189, 203, 216, 231, 245, 258, 272, 289, 303, 317, 329, 343, 355, 364

LOVING BOUNDARIES:
Days 12, 31, 56, 79, 103, 129, 153, 174, 206, 234, 269, 297, 325, 345, 360

MEAL MEDITATIONS:
Days 23, 47, 70, 93, 117, 140, 163, 187, 201, 224, 247, 271, 294, 318, 341, 365

MIDWEEK CHECK-INS:
Days 4, 11, 18, 25, 32, 39, 46, 53, 60, 67, 74, 81, 88, 95, 102, 109, 116, 123, 130, 137, 144, 151, 158, 165, 172, 179, 186, 193, 200, 207, 214, 228, 235, 242, 249, 256, 263, 271, 277, 284, 291, 298, 305, 312, 319, 326, 333, 340, 347, 354, 361

SELF-CARE:
Days 10, 30, 45, 63, 82, 100, 118, 132, 159, 173, 191, 208, 222, 238, 255, 273, 290, 306, 331, 357

SELF-COMPASSION:
Days 6, 21, 37, 54, 72, 89, 105, 121, 136, 149, 167, 182, 199, 215, 230, 243, 261, 279, 292, 307, 320, 336, 353

WEEKLY INTENTIONS:
Days 1, 8, 15, 22, 29, 36, 43, 50, 57, 64, 71, 78, 85, 92, 99, 106, 113, 120, 127, 134, 141, 148, 155, 162, 169, 176, 183, 190, 197, 204, 211, 218, 225, 232, 239, 246, 253, 260, 267, 274, 281, 288, 295, 302, 309, 316, 323, 330, 337, 344, 351, 358

Acknowledgments

This book is truly a labor of love. I wrote it during a very difficult period—in the midst of a pandemic, a global social justice uprising, and while my father was dying. I am incredibly grateful to:

- Cara Bedick, my editor, for ushering in a book I'm really proud of. Thank you for your editorial direction and extending my manuscript deadline. Thanks to the entire Chronicle Prism team. Thanks especially to Marisol Ortega for the illustrations.

- David Hale Smith, my long-time literary agent at InkWell Management Literary Agency. He not only championed this book, he was a compassionate witness to some dark days when I was unable to write.

The wisdom I share in this book is a culmination of what I learned from my patients, teachers, scientists, and thought leaders. The mistakes are all mine. I'm especially grateful to the following people:

- Daniel P. Brown, PhD
- Cynthia Price, PhD, MA, LMT
- Desiree Adaway
- Fiona Sutherland, MSc, APD, RYT
- Diane Keddy, MS, RD
- Greta Jarvis, MS
- Daniel R Siakel, PhD

- Christy Roletter
- Samantha Mullen
- Tracy Tylka, PhD
- Elyse Resch, MS, RDN, CEDRD-S
- Ryan Seay, PhD
- Andrew Huberman, PhD
- Sonalee Rashatwar, LCSW MEd

Lastly, to the Intuitive Eating professionals and Intuitive Eating community for your enthusiastic support.

Endnotes

1. Cascio, C. N., O'Donnell, M. B., Tinney, F. J., Lieberman, M. D., Taylor, S. D., Strecher, V. J., and Falk, E. B. (2016). "Self-affirmation activates brain systems associated with self-related processing and reward and is reinforced by future orientation." *Social Cognitive and Affective Neuroscience* 11 (4): 621–629, doi: 10.1093/scan/nsv136.

2. Linardon, J., and Messer, M. (2019). "My fitness pal usage in men: Associations with eating disorder symptoms and psychosocial impairment." *Eating Behavior* 33: 13–17, doi: 10.1016/j.eatbeh.2019.02.003; Levinson, C. A., Fewell, L., and Brosof, L. C. (2017). "My Fitness Pal calorie tracker usage in the eating disorders." *Eating Behavior* 27: 14–16, doi: 10.1016/j.eatbeh.2017.08.003. Accessed May 28, 2020.

3. Atlasofemotions.org.

4. Oswald, A., Chapman, J., and Wilson, C. (2017). "Do interoceptive awareness & interoceptive responsiveness mediate the relationship between body appreciation & intuitive eating in young women?" *Appetite* 109: 66–72, https://doi.org/10.1016/j.appet.2016.11.019.

5. Dweck, Carol S. *Mindset: The New Psychology of Success.* New York: Random House, 2016.

6. Adapted from the research of: Alleva, J. M., Martijn, C., Van Breukelen, G. J. P., Jansen, A., and Karos, K. (2015). "Expand Your Horizon: A programme that improves body image and reduces self-objectification by training women to focus on body functionality." *Body Image* 15: 81–89, https://doi.org/10.1016/j.bodyim.2015.07.001.

7. Krebs, P., Norcross, J. C., Nicholson, J. M., and Prochaska, J. O. (2018). "Stages of change and psychotherapy outcomes: A review and meta-analysis." *Journal of Clinical Psychology* 74 (11): 1964–1979, https://doi.org/10.1002/jclp.22683.

8. Tribole, E., and Resch, E. *Intuitive Eating*, fourth ed. New York: St. Martin's Press Essentials, 2020.

9. Lydecker, J. A., and Grilo, C. M. (2019). "Food insecurity and bulimia nervosa in the United States." *International Journal of Eating Disorders* 52 (6): 735–739; Becker, C. B., et al (2017). "Food insecurity and eating disorder pathology." *International Journal of Eating Disorders* 50: 1031–1040.

10. Schwartz, S. H. (2012). "An overview of the Schwartz Theory of Basic Values." *Online Readings in Psychology and Culture*, 2 (1).

11. Mann, T., et al (2007). "Medicare's search for effective obesity treatments: Diets are not the answer." *American Psychologist* 62 (3): 220–233; National Health and Medical Research Council. (2013). *Clinical practice guidelines for the management of overweight and obesity in adults, adolescents and children in Australia.* Melbourne: National Health and Medical Research Council, 160; O'Hara, L., and

Taylor, J. (2018). "What's wrong with the 'War on Obesity?' A narrative review of the weight-centered health paradigm and development of the 3C framework to build critical competency for a paradigm shift." *Sage Open* 8, no. 2: 2158244018772888.

[12] La Berge, A. F. (2008). "How the ideology of low fat conquered America." *Journal of the History of Medicine and Allied Sciences* 63 (2): 139–177, https://doi.org/10.1093/jhmas/jrn001.

[13] Uvnäs-Moberg, K., Handlin, L., and Petersson, M. (2015). "Self-soothing behaviors with particular reference to oxytocin release induced by non-noxious sensory stimulation." *Frontiers in Psychology* 5 (1529): 1–16.

[14] Strings, S. *Fearing the Black Body: The Racial Origins of Fat Phobia.* New York: NYU Press, 2019.

[15] Ruch, W., and Proyer, R. (2015). "Mapping strengths into virtues: The relation of the 24 VIA-strengths to six ubiquitous virtues." *Frontiers in Psychology* 6 (460): 1–12.

[16] Pinsker, J. "Something Is changing in the way people eat at home." *The Atlantic,* May 22, 2019, https://www.theatlantic.com/family/archive/2019/05/meals-couches-bedrooms-kitchen-table/590026.

[17] Allen, S. *The Science of Awe.* Berkeley: Greater Good Science Center at UC Berkeley, September 2018.

[18] "How does skin work?" *InformedHealth.org,* Cologne, Germany: Institute for Quality and Efficiency in Health Care, last updated April 11, 2019, https://www.ncbi.nlm.nih.gov/books/NBK279255; Yavorski, K. "What is the life span of skin cells?" *Sciencing.com*, updated April 5, 2019, https://sciencing.com/life-span-skin-cells-5114345.html.

[19] Communication and verification via Andrew Huberman, Ph.D., Stanford University.

[20] Lukin, K. "Toxic Positivity: Don't Always Look on the Bright Side." *Psychology Today*, August, 1, 2019, https://www.psychologytoday.com/us/blog/the-man-cave/201908/toxic-positivity-dont-always-look-the-bright-side.

[21] Laskowski, E. "What's a normal resting heart rate?" Mayo Clinic, August 29, 2018, https://www.mayoclinic.org/healthy-lifestyle/fitness/expert-answers/heart-rate/faq-20057979.

[22] See note 11.

[23] Peneau, S., Menard, E., Mejean, C., et al. (2013). "Sex and dieting modify the association between emotional eating and weight status." *American Journal of Clinical Nutrition* 97: 1307–1313, https://doi.org/10.3945/ajcn.112.054916.

[24] Rogers, C. R. *On Becoming a Person: A Therapist's View of Psychotherapy.* New York: Houghton Mifflin Publishing, 1995. Reprinted by permission of Houghton Mifflin Harcourt Publishing Company. All rights reserved.

[25] Nietzsche, F. *Thus Spoke Zarathustra: A Book for All and None*. Translated by Walter Kaufmann. New York: Modern Library, 1995, 34–35.

[26] See note 11.

[27] Mehling, W. E., Chesney, M. A., Metzler, T. J., et al. (2018). "A 12-week integrative exercise program improves self-reported mindfulness and interoceptive awareness in war veterans with posttraumatic stress symptoms." *Journal of Clinical Psychology* 74 (4): 554–565, https://doi.org/10.1002/jclp.22549.

[28] Taylor, L. *My Stroke of Insight*. New York: Penguin Publishing Group, 2008, 146. Kindle Edition.

[29] "Why electronics may stimulate you before bed." *SleepFoundation.org*, accessed May 28, 2020, https://www.sleepfoundation.org/articles/why-electronics-may-stimulate-you-bed.

[30] Turner, P., and Lefevre, C. (2017). "Instagram use is linked to increased symptoms of orthorexia nervosa." *Eating and Weight Disorders* 22: 277–284, https://doi.org/10.1007/s40519-017-0364-2.

[31] Kübler-Ross, E., and Kessler, D. *On Grief and Grieving: Finding the Meaning of Grief Through the Five Stages of Loss*. New York: Scribner, 2005.

[32] Killingsworth, M., and Gilbert D. (2010). "A wandering mind is an unhappy mind." *Science* 330 (6006): 932–932. doi: 10.1126/science.1192439.

[33] See note 24.

[34] Kale, S. "Skin hunger helps explain your desperate longing for human touch." *Wired*, April 29, 2020, https://www.wired.co.uk/article/skin-hunger-coronavirus-human-touch.

[35] Craig, A. D. (Bud). *How Do You Feel? An Interoceptive Moment with Your Neurobiolgical Self*. Princeton: Princeton University Press, 2014, 222.

[36] Holding an ice cube is a distress tolerance technique from Marsha Linehan, PhD, creator of dialectical behavior therapy, also known as DBT.

[37] Strickland, J., and Smith, M. (2014). "The anxiolytic effects of resistance exercise." *Frontiers in Psychology* 5: 753, https://doi.org/10.3389/fpsyg.2014.00753.

[38] Dolezal, L., and Lyons, B. (2017). "Health-related shame: an effective determinant of health?" *Medical Humanities* 43: 257–263.

[39] See note 11.

[40] Dana, D. . *The Polyvagal Theory in Therapy: Engaging the Rhythm of Regulation* (Norton Series on Interpersonal Neurobiology) New York: W. W. Norton & Company, 2018, 87–88.

About the Author

Evelyn Tribole, MS, RDN, **CEDRD-S** (Certified Eating Disorders Registered Dietitian-Supervisor) is the author of ten books and coauthor of the bestselling *Intuitive Eating*, a mind-body self-care eating framework with ten principles, which has given rise to over 125 studies to date, showing benefit.

As an international speaker and workshop leader, Evelyn is passionate and has been called "Wonderfully wise and funny." Evelyn enjoys training health professionals on how to help their clients cultivate a healthy relationship with food, mind, and body through the process of Intuitive Eating. To date, there are over one thousand Certified Intuitive Eating Counselors in twenty-three countries.

The media often seeks Evelyn for her expertise, and she has appeared in hundreds of interviews, including with the *New York Times*, CNN, NBC's *Today Show*, MSNBC, Fox News, *USA Today*, *The Wall Street Journal*, *The Atlantic*, *Vogue*, Ten Percent Happier, and *People* magazine. Evelyn was the nutrition expert for *Good Morning America* and a national spokesperson for the Academy of Nutrition and Dietetics for six years.

Evelyn qualified for the Olympic Trials in the first-ever women's marathon in 1984. Although she no longer competes, she is a wicked ping-pong player and avid hiker. Her favorite food is chocolate—when it can be savored slowly.